'This book is an invaluable contribution to the field of sexual abuse prevention. This book compiles insights from numerous experts who have dedicated their careers to addressing and preventing sexual abuse. It stands as an essential resource for professionals working in this challenging area of therapy, making it a highly recommended addition to their, or anyone interested in this area, bookshelves.'

Anthony Beech, *Professor (Emeritus) in Criminological Psychology*

'I am proud to be a Patron of StopSO, and equally proud of the work our therapists do to tackle the threat of child sexual abuse. The latest assessment of the number of children affected by online sexual abuse and exploitation is staggering, we are facing a global pandemic and a public health crisis. If we are to stand any hope of combatting the threat, it is going to require a whole system response. Whilst a victim focus is imperative, and one that should never be forgotten, one element of the response has to focus on working with offenders.

This book provides an invaluable insight into the complexity of the work and the challenges therapists face dealing with offenders seeking help and the impact it has on their lives and those of their families.'

Simon Bailey, *CBE, QPM, DL, MSt (Cantab) Chair of the International Policing and Public Protection Research Institute (IPPPRI)*

A Practitioner's Guide to Working with Sexual Offenders, Families, and Victims

This unique text aims to cover the many variations of presentations that a mental health professional needs to address in order to conduct effective work with sex offenders and alleged offenders, their victims, as well as their families and children.

The book is divided into three sections. It commences with an overview of the criminal justice process and its ramifications, not just for the alleged offender, but also for the wider family and friends who may feel totally out of control over what is happening in their lives, as well as for the victim. It also covers the secondary victimisation of the children of alleged offenders. The next section is designed to take some of the fear out of working with these clients, looking at unexpected specific issues that may be presented with these clients, how to address the client's trauma history, and how to support them on their journey through the criminal justice system. Chapters include working with non-offending partners, within minority groups like those within the neurodivergent or LGBTQIA+ communities, with women who commit offences, as well as with children and adolescents. Section three covers some of the therapeutic ethical dilemmas within this work, including supervision, confidentiality, safeguarding, and disclosure. Each chapter in the book is written by an experienced, hands-on therapist, giving voice and humanity to their clients.

This book is designed for all the mental health workers who find the ubiquitous issue of sexual abuse, in all its forms, coming through their office door.

Glyn Hudson-Allez, PhD, is an independent forensic psychosexual therapist who specialises in working with individuals who have sought help in respect of harmful sexual behaviours, including those who are accused of or who have committed sexual offences, using a unique integrative synthesis of neuroscience, developmental psychology, and psychodynamic therapy. She has written four books: *A Trauma-Informed Understanding of Online Offending. Adult Losses from Adolescent Searches* (2023); *Infant Losses; Adult Searches. A Neural and Developmental Perspective on Psychopathology and Sexual Offending* (2nd ed., 2011); *Sex & Sexuality. Questions and Answers for Counsellors and Psychotherapists* (2005) and *Time-Limited Therapy in a General Practice Setting: How to Help Within 6 Sessions* (1997), and has edited: *Sexual Diversity and Sexual Offending. Research, Assessment and Clinical Treatment in Psychosexual Therapy* (2014). Glyn has two fellowships: Association of Counsellors & Psychotherapists in Primary Care (CPC) and The College of Sexual and Relationship Therapists (COSRT).

A Practitioner's Guide to Working with Sexual Offenders, Families, and Victims

Demystifying Sexual Offences

Edited by Glyn Hudson-Allez

Routledge
Taylor & Francis Group
LONDON AND NEW YORK

Designed cover image: © Getty Images

First published 2025
by Routledge
4 Park Square, Milton Park, Abingdon, Oxon OX14 4RN

and by Routledge
605 Third Avenue, New York, NY 10158

Routledge is an imprint of the Taylor & Francis Group, an informa business

British Library Cataloguing-in-Publication Data
A catalogue record for this book is available from the British Library

ISBN: 978-1-032-83387-3 (hbk)
ISBN: 978-1-032-83384-2 (pbk)
ISBN: 978-1-003-50910-3 (ebk)

DOI: 10.4324/9781003509103

Typeset in Times New Roman
by Apex CoVantage, LLC

Contents

List of Contributors

Clare S. Allely is a Professor of Forensic Psychology at the University of Salford in England and is an affiliate member of the Gillberg Neuropsychiatry Centre at Gothenburg University, Sweden. Clare is an Honorary Research Fellow in the College of Medical, Veterinary and Life Sciences affiliated to the Institute of Health and Wellbeing at the University of Glasgow. Clare acts as an expert witness in criminal cases involving defendants with autism spectrum disorder and contributes to the evidence base used in the courts on psychology and legal issues through her published work. She is the author of *The Psychology of Extreme Violence: A Case Study Approach to Serial Homicide, Mass Shooting, School Shooting and Lone-actor Terrorism* (2020) and *Autism Spectrum Disorder in the Criminal Justice System: A Guide to Understanding Suspects, Defendants and Offenders with Autism* (2022).

Emma Barwell is a registered Social Worker, with 20 years' experience of working with children and families. Alongside Independent Assessment work, Emma delivers training for the Centre of Expertise on Child Sexual Abuse and psycho-education programmes for the Lucy Faithfull Foundation. Emma is trained in Psychodynamic Counselling and applies this in her therapeutic interventions with those who harm and have caused harm to others.

Joan Birkmyre began her career in Nursing working in Medical Research, Occupational Health and Teaching in Higher and Further Education (Health & Social Care and Counselling). Her counselling career began in Relate in 1988 alongside doing a BA degree with the Open University. She worked for Relate N.I. as a Marital and Couples Counsellor and Psychosexual Therapist, and subsequently as part of the training team. She is currently in private practice and is a therapist and supervisor. Her specialist subject areas include sexual compulsive behaviour as co-founder of ATSAC (Association for the Treatment of Sexual Addiction and Compulsivity) and Sexual Offending as a registered member of StopSO.

Dana Braithwaite is a COSRT Senior Accredited Sexual and Relationship Psychotherapist and Senior Accredited Supervisor, specialising in forensic psychosexual therapy. She is a co-founder of StopSO UK, former Chair and Trustee of

StopSO. She is currently vice chair of COSRT (College of Sexual and Relationship Therapists), where she has been a Trustee for the last nine years. She is also qualified to work with sexually compulsive behaviours. Dana has a successful private practice and is the Clinical Lead for a Psychosexual Service with 30 years' experience in the NHS. She ran a CPD training programme for the University of Central Lancashire on forensic sexual offending.

John Goss is a counsellor and supervisor who specialises in working with men who have committed sexual offences and those with compulsive sexual behaviours. John identifies as being gay and has lots of experience in working with LGBTQIA+ clients, which compliments his work when sexual offending and compulsive sexual behaviours are presented.

Matthew Graham is a practising solicitor and partner operating nationally in criminal justice. With extensive frontline experience over more than two decades, Matthew brings his practical, realistic approach to both practice in the criminal justice system and in safeguarding work, including supporting other rehabilitation and intervention professionals. Matthew works with individuals and organisations across the public, private, charitable, and third sector to share and enhance best practice.

Trudy Hannington is the Senior Psychosexual Therapist who leads a team of five psychosexual therapists at the Leger clinic in Doncaster, South Yorkshire, England. She has worked in sexual health for over 25 years and specialised as a psychosexual therapist since 2002 after training at the Porterbrook Clinic at Sheffield. She is a Senior Accredited member, Supervisor, Fellow and former Chair of COSRT (College for Sex & Relationship Therapists), and is one of the co-founders of StopSO.

Glyn Hudson-Allez is a BPS Chartered Psychologist who has worked as a therapist for nearly 40 years, eight of which were in Primary Health Care, latterly specialising in working with people who have diverse or potentially deviant sexual behaviour, using her unique therapeutic style of integrating attachment theory and neuroscientific research. She has published five books: *Time Limited Therapy in a General Practice Setting* (1997); *Sex & Sexuality: Questions and Answers for Counsellors and Psychotherapists* (2005); *Infant Losses; Adult Searches. A Neural and Developmental Perspective on Psychopathology and Sexual Offending* (2011, now in its second edition), *A Trauma-Informed Understanding of Online Offending. Adult Losses from Adolescent Searches* (2023), and her edited book, *Sexual Diversity and Sexual Offending. Research, Assessment and Clinical Treatment in Psychosexual Therapy* (2014). For four years Glyn was a Trustee of the charity Specialist Treatment Organisation for the Perpetrators and Victims of Sexual Offending (StopSO UK). Glyn has two professional fellowships: the Association of Counsellors & Psychotherapists in Primary Care (CPC), and The College for Sexual and Relationship Therapy (COSRT).

Sue Maxwell trained as a nurse in general and mental health and subsequently trained as a relationship and psychosexual therapist in the 1980s. She worked in the NHS for 30 years, latterly as nurse manager in the community mental health service for people with HIV and AIDS. More recently, Sue worked with Relationships Scotland (RS) as Joint Head of Network Services retiring in 2013. For 23 years Sue has worked in private practice offering psychotherapy to clients couples and families. She supervises private therapists, NHS psychosexual therapists, ATSAC therapists working with sexual compulsivity and StopSO therapists seeing clients with out-of-control sexual behaviours that breach the Sex Offences Act. She is currently on the Board of Trustees of StopSO.

Antounette Philippides was a Probation Officer for 32 years, working in Birmingham, West Midlands. She held a number of posts within the organisation, including working in prisons and mental health teams. Her cases have been primarily from the high and very high risk of causing harm MAPPA offenders, including working with sexual offenders. She retrained as a psychotherapist and now works as a therapist in private practice. She joined StopSO in 2019, became a Trustee, and then Chair in 2022.

Ian Richards originally studied Person Centred Counselling & Psychotherapy, obtaining a Degree at the University of Warwick in 2015. He is a qualified sex addiction therapist and has been working with StopSO since 2017.

Michael Sheath worked as a Probation Officer for ten years prior to spending 25 years with The Lucy Faithfull Foundation, a charity specialising in preventing child sexual abuse. Whilst there he acted as an expert witness in family court proceedings, and developed a specialism in training police officers and social workers in understanding the mindset of men who view child sexual abuse material. He is employed as a trainer on the Europol online sexual exploitation course, and for CEPOL, the European Police College. He is the author of a play addressing trauma and secondary trauma in child sexual abuse material investigations, entitled *Crossing the Line.*

Dr Andrew Smith has worked in the area of sexual offending as an expert witness in the UK for 21 years, first with Ray Wyre Associates, then full-time with the Lucy Faithfull Foundation from 2006 until 2015. He was awarded a PhD by Cardiff University in 2010 for research on strengths-based approaches to sex offending, and is a regular contributor to journals and books. He is a qualified probation officer and counsellor. He regularly trains therapists to work with individuals posing a sexual risk for StopSO (Specialist Treatment Organisation for Perpetrators and Survivors of Sexual Offending). He has published two books: *Counselling Male Sexual Offenders: A Strengths-Focused Approach* (2017) and *Counselling Partners and Relatives of Individuals who have Sexually Offended: A Strengths-Focused Eclectic Approach* (2022).

Michael Stock is a therapist working private practice. He has a BSc and MSc in Statistics, a Certificate in Counselling, a postgraduate diploma in Psychosexual Therapy, a Professional Certificate in Therapeutic Practice with Sex Offenders and a Diploma in Individual and Group Supervision.

Tom Taylor MBACP (Accred) is a UK-registered psychotherapist in private practice, specialising in psychological trauma, sexualised trauma, and compulsive sexual behaviour. He has worked with a forensic client group for over ten years and been a member of StopSO since 2014.

Terri Van-Leeson is a Consultant Forensic Psychologist with 26 years' experience in the field of psychology spanning a wide range of services and roles, now working in private practice. Terri worked with men convicted of serious sexual offences in custodial settings and was always struck by the high levels of sexual trauma the majority of these men had experienced during childhood. Her passion for prevention has seen Terri working increasingly with children in the community who have suffered varying degrees of sexual abuse, and who have become sexually reactive, presenting with problematic harmful sexual behaviour.

Louise Wilcox is a psychodynamically-trained registered Social Worker with 30 years' experience. Her experience spans child protection, generic social work, and emergency social work. She now works in the faith and charity sector.

Preface: Walking a tightrope alongside those who cross the line

Glyn Hudson-Allez

There is now burgeoning literature demonstrating that individuals in the UK being arrested and subsequently convicted of online sexual offences is reaching epidemic proportions since the 2019–20 Covid pandemic (Centre of Expertise, 2023; Grant, 2023). The NSPCC (2024) have argued that there is a 79% increase in recorded offences between 2017/18 and 2022/2023. These arrests, colloquially known as 'The Knock', precipitate mental health breakdown and suicidal ideation in the alleged offender, and secondary traumatisation for their families and children, as well as traumatisation for the victims (these issues are dealt with thoroughly in this book). The consequence is that vast numbers of these (predominantly) men, their victims, and their families are seeking psychological and therapeutic support, often at the recommendation of the police, their solicitor, or their GP. There is no state-organised facility for these individuals to turn to; they are all essentially left to deal with the ramifications alone. Therefore, many seek support from counsellors, therapists, and psychologists who may have a limited understanding of the therapeutic specialism required to deal with a person who is embarked on the journey through the Criminal Justice System (CJS), or who fear they will. As such, many therapists have preconceived ideas about 'sex offenders' and their potential danger to the community, making them judgmental within the therapy room. Therapists may struggle with the work, or even reject the person altogether. Rejection might alienate and push the individual underground, leading to further potential offences. As therapy with these individuals is a child protection issue, the more knowledge and understanding of the aetiology and rehabilitative treatment we can provide, the less risk there will be to the victims, the clients themselves, their families, as well as the public at large. This book has been designed to offer knowledge and support to these professional mental health workers, to give them confidence to undertake what at times can be very challenging work.

The Specialist Treatment Organisation for Perpetrators and Survivors of Sexual Offending (StopSO UK) is a child-protection charity offering access to specialist therapists trained to work with people who may have compulsive thoughts or behaviours that may lead them into forbidden territory, most commonly viewing pornography online or communicating in chat rooms. They also have trained forensic therapists to work with those who have been arrested for crossing the line into committing a contact sexual offence, and those who have been convicted and are post-sentence. They provide support and help for the families of the people who have committed an offence, and specialist treatment for their victims.

> Seeing a StopSO counsellor means having the support of someone who is impartial and non-judgemental, who can help me to make the changes needed to turn my life around and make myself into a better person, making sure that my behaviour stays in the past and does not cause any more harm to other people.
>
> ('J', a StopSO client)

Established in 2012, with its mission statement to prevent the first crime, StopSO now have over 100 independent therapists working throughout England, Scotland, Wales, and Northern Ireland, who are trained and qualified to work with this client group. The organisation has a varied training programme to keep up to date with latest trends and to offer best practice to the clients that self-refer to the organisation. Since its inception, StopSO therapists have worked with hundreds of individuals and as a result have prevented potential or further abuse of children.

Knowing that the provision that StopSO members provide is only the tip of the iceberg in terms of a nationwide need, senior members of the organisation and their colleagues have contributed to this book, generously offering their knowledge and expertise to those who may be struggling with a client before them. It aims to cover many of the variations of presentations that counsellors and therapists need to address in order to conduct effective work with these clients, written by experienced practitioners in the field. It is designed for all mental health workers who find the ubiquitous issue of sexual abuse, in all its forms, come through their consulting room door.

Working with individuals who have committed a sexual offence can be challenging. Schwartz *et al.* eloquently argued:

> All of us have been perpetrators of some kind, at some level, either toward self or other. All of us have been victims of deliberate or inadvertent perpetration . . . Even the darkest perpetrators carry a light inside them, albeit buried under decades or generations of traumatic experience. Are we not, as healers, responsible for holding the belief that everyone has the potential to be healed? . . . It is important for therapists, as well as clients, to address their experiences as a perpetrator, as well as a victim, in order for integrated healing to occur in its totality . . . This work is part and parcel of addressing distressing events that are experienced internally as well as in the context of external relationships. Avoiding this aspect of our history does a disservice to one's self as therapists as well as preventing important, holistic work from being done with clients.
>
> (Schwartz *et al.* 2017, p. 76)

Friedman (1988) suggested that we need to accept our client on their own terms, whilst also refusing to settle for those terms. This is especially true for an offender.

Wallin (2007) points out that our clients are capable of more feeling, thoughtful-ness, connection, and initiative than they believe they are, and it is our role to help them find the right balance for them to change whilst staying the same; if we expect too little of them, they may feel betrayed; expect too much and their vulnerabilities may go unrecognised.

This book comprises three sections.

Section 1 The knock and its consequences

Whether the person has had 'the knock', that is, a visit from the police to inform of a potential prosecution, or feel that they might, or a partner who has discovered something unacceptable on their loved-one's computer or phone, in Chapter 1 Tom Taylor and Glyn Hudson-Allez try to answer some of the questions and anxieties that are raised in the therapy room. Why do they do it? What leads them to cross the line in such unacceptable ways? They argue that the current social and criminal processes that occur after the knock, rather than ameliorating the problem, create such alienation and hate against the offenders that it contributes to their suicidal-ity and makes recidivism more likely. Antounette Philippides in Chapter 2, speaks on behalf of the victims; whether they are victims from physical sexual abuse in the present or historically, or victims of the online imagery or chat, and also for the wider family and friends who may feel totally out of control over what is hap-pening in their lives. Clients who have been arrested often present with fear and anxiety about what the future holds for them, for their relationship, and for their children. Michael Sheath in Chapter 3, outlines the damage caused by the second-ary traumatisation to the wives and children of those arrested, feeling their world is falling down around them, becoming the innocent victims of the criminal justice system (CJS), and how society responds to them. In Chapter 4, Emma Barwell and Louise Wilcox provide an understanding of the child protection procedures follow-ing an arrest from a social worker perspective. Why do they stop men who have 'just' viewed child sexual abuse material (CSAM) online having access to their own children? Finally, for those unfamiliar with the CJS process for people who commit sexual offences, Glyn Hudson-Allez outlines in Chapter 5 the 'long and winding road' from the police investigation, the court process, and the probation re-quirements post-conviction. In the final chapter in this section, Chapter 6, Michael Stock uses his statistical skills to demonstrate how ubiquitous this presentation has become and makes a comparison between national data and a small sample of questionnaires from StopSO clients.

Section 2 Working with the variety of presentations: not a one-size-fits-all approach

This section is designed to take some of the fear out of working with these clients, to explain to counsellors and therapists that reading about the topic and with good supervision, they can do good work helping these clients turn their lives around.

It advocates addressing each client as an individual, looking at the client's trauma history, and supporting them through the fear of their journey through the CJS with their individual presentations, rather than using the one-size-fits-all approach to sexual offenders common to probation-run treatment programmes. In Chapter 7, Ian Richards discusses the compulsive/addictive side of the use of pornography, potentiated by dopamine in the neural pathways and underpinned by repetition compulsion from adverse childhood experiences. Why are some people drawn to sexually acting out? What does that say about their sexual template, and where do addictive or compulsive mechanisms come into play? In Chapter 8, Trudy Hannington, one of the founder members of StopSO, talks about working with the secondary trauma of the non-offending partners/wives/husbands, who are often left reeling with more questions than answers. She explores some of the reasons why women make the decision to stay with their partners and what therapists can do to support, rather than judge, that decision. Of course, not all partners are women, so in Chapter 9, John Goss focuses on members of the gay community, who can have a different outlook toward sexual diversity. In particular, John discusses the issue of consent given through social media compared to that of real life, and whether those enjoying chemsex are in a position to verify consent. Terri Van-Leeson, in Chapter 10, discusses the younger clients referred to StopSO, who have engaged in unhealthy, potentially socially- or boundary-violating sexual behaviour, some who have been as young as six years old. She outlines two distinct profiles of child clients: the first are children who have a known sexual trauma history of their own, having been sexually abused. The second are children with a pre-existing diagnosis of learning difficulties and/or high functioning autism spectrum disorder (hfASD), on which Clare Allely elaborates in Chapter 11 for adult presentations, with their innate characteristics that can lead them to unwittingly commit sexual offending behaviour online. In Chapter 12, Glyn Hudson-Allez discusses the prevalence of women committing sexual offences, which is very small compared to those of men, but seems to be rising. Why would this be, and what allows women to venture down a path that seems like an anathema to society? The section ends with Chapter 13, in which Andrew Smith discusses the training requirements of therapeutic working with people who commit sexual offences, in particular how counsellors can emotionally manage the demands of working with such a stigmatised group, and how the particular shame associated with sex offenders can sometimes be vicariously felt by counsellors themselves, in terms of fears about reputational damage. Andrew explores how training counsellors/therapists to reflect upon and make explicit their often complex, motivations for working with this client group, prevents empathy from tipping over into collusion.

Section 3 Thorny issues

This section covers many of the complex issues that are raised from therapists experienced in this kind of work, particularly regarding supervision, confidentiality, safeguarding and disclosure, some of which may be legal but not ethical, and others ethical but not legal (Hudson-Allez, 2004). Sue Maxwell, in Chapter 14, argues for the importance of good supervision when working with these clients, and that means supervisors who know and understand forensic work, and how supervisors help therapists maintain resilience and compassion for their work and to prevent vicarious trauma from this specific client load. In Chapter 15, Dana Braithwaite, another founder member of StopSO, discusses a therapeutic approach to risk assessment and management, increasing therapeutic skills and confidence. Unlike the safeguarding measures discussed in Chapter 4, Dana outlines the dilemma of the lone therapist, who has a different set of pressures and responsibilities to maintain therapeutic boundaries, to build trust with the client, revealing often unconscious processes which may affect safeguarding issues, not just currently, but considering future safeguarding issues for the client and their families to help prevent him from re-offending. In Chapter 16, Matthew Graham, a solicitor experienced with these types of clients, offers an understanding of the legal framework regarding disclosure, the factors that need weighing when considering disclosure, and the practical steps for a practitioner to consider. In balancing potentially competing public interests whilst maintaining trusting, confidential relationships with clients, the principles of safeguarding and public protection can be viewed through the lens of harm reduction, bringing structure and confidence to an aspect of practice often perceived as a minefield. Finally, one of the most common reasons given by therapists unwilling to see clients who have committed a sexual offence is the fear of having to write letters or reports for the courts, so in Chapter 17, Terri Van-Leeson and Glyn Hudson-Allez offer help in formulating these. Where the requirements may differ from England and Wales, Sue Maxwell highlights the differences in Scotland and Joan Birkmyre presents the case from Northern Ireland. The last word, in Chapter 18, goes to a client, 'Matt', who wanted to share his experience, hoping that others might take note and learn from it. Never a day goes by when he doesn't regret what he has done.

Each chapter author has represented their professional opinion from their experience of working with this client presentation in a respectful, honest, and comprehensive way, being open and generous in their knowledge and understanding of the topics covered. They wish to encourage more therapists to take up the mantle and help with a tsunami of referrals, particularly from online offenders. Veronique Valliere argues:

> It takes a special type of professional who wants to work with a sexual offender. I am grateful whenever I find one or meet one who is interested in genuinely doing the hard work it takes. It is important to remember that you are working with people who have a level of deviance that changed their relationship with the world so that they risked everything to hurt someone, in pursuit of gratification. Working with people who have done this requires the ability to see the world and others for what it is, to recognise danger and face the realities these

offenders present boldly. If you can do this and do it properly, you are doing something important that helps not only the offender, but your community.

(Valliere, 2023, p. 125)

I believe StopSO therapists are these special types of professionals.

References

Centre of Expertise on Child Sexual Abuse (2023) *Managing risk and trauma after online sexual offending.* csacentre.org.uk/research-resources/practice-resources/managing-risk-and-trauma-after-online-sexual-offending/.

Friedman, L. (1988) The Anatomy of Psychotherapy. Analytic Press.

Grant, H. (2023, 4 December) Thousands of UK young people caught watching online child abuse images. *The Guardian.*

Hudson-Allez, G. (2004) Threats to psychotherapeutic confidentiality: Can psychotherapists in the UK really offer a confidentiality ethic to their clients? *Psychodynamic Practice,* 10(3), 317–331.

NSPCC (2024) As child abuse image crimes increase, we're calling for Ofcom and tech companies to take action. https://www.nspcc.org.uk/about-us/news-opinion/2024/Child-abuse-image-crimes-increase-calling-ofcom-tech-companies-take-action/.

Schwartz, L., Corrigan, F., Hull, A. & Raju, R. (2017) *The Comprehensive Resource Model. Effective therapeutic techniques for the healing of complex trauma.* Routledge.

Valliere, V. N. (2023) *Unmasking the Sexual Offender.* Routledge.

Wallin, D. J. (2007) *Attachment in Psychotherapy.* Guilford Press.

Section 1

The knock and its consequences

Chapter 1

When worlds collide

The secret lives and everyday lives of perpetrators of online sexual offenders, clashing with the devastating reality of the knock!

Tom Taylor and Glyn Hudson-Allez

Introduction

The meteoric rise of the internet and the accessibility and anonymity it provides (Cooper, 2013) has facilitated an ideal forum for an increasingly disillusioned, lonely and isolated population here in the UK to seek such things as escapism, distraction, excitement, connection and solace. Social media use, online gaming, chat forums and online pornography all represent extremely common uses of the worldwide web that have become cultural pastimes in their own right. Such relationships with the internet are growing at an exponential rate (Christiansen, 2023), and shows no visible signs of abating.

For perpetrators of online sexual offences, this virtual environment provides ample opportunity to create and engage with a part of themselves that they are able to separate and keep hidden from their everyday existence with relative ease. This means that friends, family, partners and colleagues remain oblivious to their 'hidden lives', until the knock on the door (the police), culminating in a collision of previously disconnected and compartmentalised areas of their lives, resulting in devastating consequences of existential proportions. Obviously illegal internet use does not happen in a vacuum. This chapter will outline and discuss common themes that perpetrators experience following the knock, as their lives, relationships and everyday realities implode. The process will be explored within the context of a range of potential predisposing, causal and maintenance factors, which all have significant meaning for understanding and treating online offending behaviours, whilst promoting the overall aim of protecting children and vulnerable members of society.

The scope of the problem

Listening to clients on a daily basis, as they discuss, recount and explain their current difficulties, what one realises is how reactive modern life is. How much of our daily experiences: the responsibilities we each struggle with, including bills to pay, children to get to school on time, husbands, wives, partners and/or older family members that we have to worry about and/or take care of, are merely things that we

DOI: 10.4324/9781003509103-2

struggle with silently, and without consciously thinking about very much. Perhaps this is one of the many reasons why more Eastern philosophical practices and ways of being, such as mindfulness and yoga, which place emphasis on becoming more in the present moment and grounded within us (Kabat-Zinn, 2019) have witnessed an upsurge in popularity over the preceding decades. Because such concepts and ideas both acknowledge and highlight the varying levels of disconnect that many of us experience and struggle with daily.

There is a sad irony in the fact that, in a modern world where technological advancements have enabled us to have a wealth of devices and means of communicating with others regardless of geographical distance, perhaps more people feel isolated, alone and disconnected than ever. It is of course impossible to ponder such thoughts without considering the significant role that the internet has played in this phenomenon. The power of connection is indeed a life-affirming, and ultimately meaningful, experience. As social animals, we are hardwired for connection to such an extent that as evolution dictates, we literally cannot, nor will not, survive without attachment (Panksepp & Biven, 2021).

Whilst watching an interview with the comedian Jimmy Carr (2024), he discussed his confusion and frustration at the claim that, when people are feeling unhappy with who they are, or that their lives have not panned out as they expected or anticipated, people just move somewhere else and reinvent themselves, be anyone they want to be, and live their lives as that person instead. This form of escapism may be a nice idea for many to consider, and for some it may even be a viable option. However, for most of us, the reality of such an extreme endeavour is simply unattainable and unrealistic. Upon reflection though, in many ways, the internet has provided an alternative world and space where such things are not so unrealistic and much more attainable. Consider the power of social media, where millions of people post information and details of their lives every day, that in many cases may be dubious at best, and literally untrue at their worst. Who has not considered the fantasy of being someone else, or living someone else's life? The internet has provided an alternative universe and reality where the possibilities are literally infinite. It has also provided a separate reality, safe from the reality of daily life. However, the reality of everyday life comes back to bite the individual who has gone too far and crossed the line into offending online, which often leads to a knock from the police serving as a huge wake-up call.

The experiences of perpetrators following the knock

For most of us it is difficult, if not impossible, to imagine what it feels like to receive the knock on the door from the police, specifically for illegal online behaviour. From that moment, their lives quite literally implode, leading to states of fear, terror, shame, guilt and consequently a sense of their lives suddenly feeling in complete freefall. One client's description of such an experience was expressed as 'I feel as if the arse has fallen out of my world'. When everything we know, everything we have created, care about or matters to us and represents meaning in our lives is under threat, we are ultimately catapulted into existential crisis territory. If everything we have accumulated feels lost and/or unattainable, then we, by definition, may feel as if we have nothing else to lose. When we feel that we have nothing to lose, we are at our most dangerous in terms of risk, both to ourselves and/or to others, which is why suicidality with this client group is so high.

It is both interesting and concerning then, that following the knock on the door, the slow, lumbering legal process that follows involves isolating the alleged perpetrator from everything in their lives that they care about. If they have children, they are forced to leave their homes and find alternative accommodation. Husbands, wives and/or partners, particularly when co-parenting children, are often actively advised and encouraged by professionals to leave their life partners. Those under investigation often lose their jobs, careers and friends as well as their families once this hurricane hits. It feels important to note at this point, that when taking the morality, the 'right and wrong' regarding the nature of the offences either alleged or committed, out of the equation and viewing this process purely via a risk assessment offense reduction and management lens, that this entire process is significantly flawed. If one considers any individual who may be deemed a risk to society within any given context, and taking everything they have away from them, then forcing them to live their lives in isolation, shame, depression, guilt and self-loathing, it does nothing to reduce risk, but increases it significantly. The risks then increase even more if the media, either newspapers, online news or social media, report on the convictions, dehumanising the offenders as 'monsters', 'pedos' and 'perverts', you thus have a recipe for the five steps to group hate (Reicher, Haslam & Rath, 2008):

1. identifying the ingroup (us),
2. excluding the outgroup (them),
3. elaborating the threat from them,
4. championing the good in virtuous us,
5. celebrating the eradication of them

A powerful, destructive process, dividing communities and destroying lives.

Working with the presentation, trauma, and attachment-informed practice

Attachment theory has been predominant in psychological theory since the observational studies of John Bowlby (1988). However, Allan Schore (1994) argued that there was a physiological process that underpins our need to attach, which led neuroscientists to investigate further. We now understand that human babies are born with seven pre-programmed neurological circuits, six of which are designed for attachment for survival of the infant, with the seventh (the sex template) coming later for survival of the species (Panksepp, 1998; Hudson-Allez, 2011). These attachment neural pathways encourage the child and the mother to visually communicate with each other, and in doing so, the emotional centres of the infant's brain start to develop emotional awareness. If, for whatever reason, infants do not get the care that they seek, fear of rejection and abandonment creates a threat to life, so the secure attachment circuitry is bypassed, and a secondary pathway is developed. This is a survival strategy for the infant, and manifests in insecure attachment behaviours, most commonly described as preoccupation, avoidance or ambivalence, and forms the behavioural attachment template for relationships for the developing child with their peers, and later in their adult relationships. Painful things happen to many of us as children. If we are in a secure environment, we can build resilience and resourcefulness through the coregulation of our attachment figures to cope with the adversity. But if we start life with an insecure attachment, we become disconnected and split, and the pain becomes a wound that festers. Insecure attachment distorts everything.

Insecure attachment is a predisposing factor in our understanding of our work with online offenders, who most commonly will have an avoidant attachment style: they fear closeness and intimacy with another person in case their needs are not met, so tend to retreat within themselves, or to seek comfort from less threatening environments. The internet offers a perfect place to have sex without intimacy, intensity and desire without threat; pornography will never reject or abandon, and will always offer more.

We incorporate an attachment focus with all of our clinical practice, as we believe it holds profound meaning not only for the therapeutic relationship itself, but also for our understanding of ourselves in relation to others. Additionally, our attachment template can represent significant potential predisposing and maintenance factors in repeated patterns, behaviours and relational processes, including sexuality and compulsive behaviours. Having an initial understanding of our client's attachment style represents an extremely useful starting point for clinical assessment and case formulation which may then be used to inform treatment (Hudson-Allez, 2023). As Schwartz and Southern (2017) propose, sexual compulsivity is generally more to do with attachment, intimacy and connection with self and others, rather than sex.

Trauma

Another predisposing issue in this client demographic is a history of trauma. Much is made of the argument that only a third of individuals (Johnson et al., 2018) who commit a sexual offence were sexually abused in their own childhood or adolescence, thus rejecting any correlation between the two. However, Ogloff et al. (2012) conducted a 45-year follow-up study and found that childhood victims of sexual abuse were almost five times more likely than the general population to be charged with any offence than their non-abused counterparts, with the strongest correlations found for sexual and violent offences. Similarly, those who had experienced childhood abuse were more likely to become further victims of crimes of a sexual or violent nature. Many online offenders find themselves drawn to watching online a re-enactment of what happened to them in their own history, and until they have worked through their own abuse trauma in therapy, they often do not have the head space to consider empathy toward the victims they see repeatedly online. Some clients, particularly those who are neurodiverse (see Chapter 11), have delayed social and developmental issues, and engage in sexual curiosity online revisiting past issues but getting developmentally stuck, most commonly at an adolescent phase.

Childhood trauma is a recognised predisposing factor in mental health presentations, and it is also a precipitating factor in the clients that we see. However, as Gabor and Daniel Maté (2024) argued, trauma is not an event *per se*, with a rating scale of extreme traumatic events down to mild innocuous events, but how the child or adult experienced it within themselves. Life events as a child, adolescent or as an adult can have detrimental effects on the individual, whether it is bereavement and loss, domestic coercion and/or violence, serious road traffic accidents, etc. (it is rare for someone to have only one traumatic event, there is usually an accumulation of them), all of which produce an existential anxiety regarding our own safety and mortality. And, of course, the knock, of itself, is a traumatic life event, for the alleged offender and for his wife or partner, children and extended family, which will be discussed in more detail in Chapter 3.

As mentioned, trauma in our client's childhood is not just about violence and/ or abuse. Using an attachment frame, loss is a significant trauma to child who later, in adolescence or adulthood, find that they 'act out', as they cannot resolve the emotional conflicts that have materialised. Judith Lewis Herman (1992) identified traumatic events that generally are a threat to life or bodily integrity, which produces feeling of helplessness, hopelessness, loss of control and a fear of annihilation (which links back to attachment and the need to survive), which can recondition the nervous system into hyper-aroused and hypervigilant states. These states not only persist during the day, but also affect the individual's sleep patterns, taking longer to fall asleep, being more sensitive to background noise and being more likely to wake frequently during the night. During these times, technology has provided an answer: the oblivion provided by constantly searching the web for prolonged periods in a trance-like fugue state, lying in bed with the smart phone, not mindful of the person lying next to them, or sneaking off into a separate room to use the iPad or laptop.

Stephen Porges (2017) considers that trauma is a chronic disruption of connectedness in relationships. That it is impossible to live a joyful life with another whilst feeling unsafe, due to polyvagal shutdown of the autonomic nervous system, which is shaped and regulated through interactions with others whom we care about. Trauma also damages and distorts our relationship with ourselves, with those we love and with the world. As psychotherapists, we work with relationships. We have a passionate belief in the healing, and transformative effects of connection (attachment) and attunement in the therapeutic relationship, which is generally missing from the lives most of the clients that we work with. When we think about the cultural and social stigmas associated with any sexual crime, let alone those involving children, they generally evoke feelings of disgust and revulsion for many. Such visceral reactions are certainly understandable in many respects, as for the majority within society, the idea of vulnerable children being sexually exploited and/or harmed in any way are ultimately intolerable and abhorrent. However, our societal expectations facilitate a blame culture, where people project their adversity onto others, unwilling to take responsibility for their own projections and agency in an event.

Therefore, it is vital, as a therapist, to be completely present for the offender in a non-judgemental way. We need to be obligated to provide for them a corrective attachment experience in a way that other people maybe do not want or cannot do, using a trauma-informed approach. We use Carl Rogers' (1977) core conditions of client-centred therapy: genuineness, congruence, empathetic understanding and unconditional positive regard. We give them what people needed as babies: PACE: playfulness, acceptance, curiosity and empathy (Golding & Hughes, 2012). We argue that these offenders need it more than many other clients because everyone else seems to hate them, and they hate themselves too. This Rogerian way of being in the therapy room is necessary for rehabilitation, but of course, not sufficient for offending work to take place, but first the client needs to build trust in therapeutic attachment; that they will not be rejected or abandoned. They can then start to reduce their shame, because the therapeutic alliance makes them feel safe; providing a safe base.

When working with clients holding on to trauma, we use Herman's (1992) three stages of recovery model adapted by her former student Janina Fisher (2021): stabilising the physical and emotional sensations to create a safe and stable 'here and now'; overcoming the fear of the trauma to come to terms with it (Eye-Movement Desensitisation Reprocessing Therapy (EMDR; Shapiro, 2018) may be useful at this stage); and integrating and moving on, to develop a greater capacity for attachment and focusing on personal and professional goals. This is a collaborative process with the client, rather than them being a passive recipient of therapy, where we provide a lot of psychoeducation about the physiological and neurological ramifications of trauma to help them understand its manifestations, always with plenty of emotional support.

Sexual compulsivity and sexual addiction

A maintaining factor in the route to offending is the neurological dopamine hit from sexually acting out (see Chapter 7). This might be online masturbatory 'edging' for hours at a time, whether it is viewing pornographic imagery or going into chat rooms for sexual conversations or live web-cam sex. Or it may be having affairs, one-night stands, visiting sex workers, or experimenting with alternative sexual experiences outside of one's own sexuality. Dopamine precipitates this seeking process: 'wanting' more. On the face of it, as sex-positive psychotherapists, there is nothing wrong with this behaviour, providing it all occurs within the boundaries of consenting adults. However, if the behaviour becomes compulsive, it can interfere with daily living and long-term relationships when it is conducted in secret without the partner's knowledge. This is where an individual will describe themselves as being split; having two sides of themselves: one side being an ordinary family man in a long-term relationship, the other being a dark and secretive side (shadow) producing huge feelings of guilt and shame.

The concept of the shadow represents a focal factor in Carl Jung's (1957) model of the human psyche and something he wrote about extensively throughout his life and career. Jung both understood, and knew all too well, that the shadow represents those parts of ourselves that we may recognise as too difficult to recognise and acknowledge. '*It is usually the most devalued, inferior, repulsive, animal part of ourselves, which remains mostly dark and unknown*' (Mahmoud, 2023, p.16). For many of the men who have committed online sexual offences, they are already familiar with their shadow, whether consciously or subconsciously. Depression, anxiety, shame, guilt, loneliness, isolation, loss, hopelessness, failure and/or fear of failure, are all relevant examples of clients' trajectory leading into online offending behaviour. The web offers the comfort they are seeking, but they will never find.

If the seeking for more sexual stimulation escalates from boredom or habituation into needing greater variety and intensity, an itch that can never be scratched, then this suggests the compulsive behaviour has become addictive (Maté, 2018; Hudson-Allez, 2023). This is where the person is in danger of crossing the line into illegal territory on a pathway that they cannot stop. Not everyone who looks at child sexual abuse material (CSAM) online are sexually aroused by children. Some are, but many can be horrified by it, but still cannot stop looking, just as the 'looky-loos' or 'rubber-neckers' slowing down at a motorway crash in the hope of seeing some blood and gore. Some online viewers are turned on by the children they see, especially if they have been abused, neglected, or treated with contempt themselves.

Many clients identify themselves as pornography addicts in their first session of therapy, often having used adult pornography from early teenage years. They minimise the activity as 'what blokes do' without realising it is damaging their sexual script, and causing confusion and anxiety over their sexuality. They get 'plugged in' to the internet, being reactive in their thoughts and feelings, providing the ultimate escape from life. Certainly, pornography does contribute to the desensitisation of images viewed online, needing to see more to get the same stimulus, and they will compartmentalise this need from their real life. It is not until they get the wake-up call from the knock that the deep guilt and shame, already present in huge amounts, debilitates and breaks down their mental health.

Shame

In the societal construct of unacceptable offences, what ranks highest is sexual offences against children. Yet the offender is also part of the society who perceives such offences as unforgivable. Thus, the split person on one level hates and vilifies himself for his own behaviour, creating palpable shame that he wears on his sleeve. The other, dark side will minimise and argue that they didn't know it was wrong, that the images were not real, and that the conversations were merely fantasy. Yet they do know it is wrong; and the shame of being unable to stop is reinforced and maintained through the dopamine in the brain that it uses and produces.

It is important for any therapist who is either already doing this type of work, or indeed those who are considering it, to identify the predisposing contribution of traumatic shame of the client and also to acknowledge and acquaint ourselves of our own shame, notwithstanding valid arguments that any psychotherapeutic work with clients who are struggling with issues in their own lives will inevitably bring us therapists into confrontation and/or contact with the territory of our own shame. Specialised psychosexual work leads us into shameful territory because of the cultural and social messages that we all receive regarding sex; this predisposes us into associating anything sexual with shame. Most of us will be familiar with those people who literally say the word sex, and/or refer to anything sexual, maybe blushing and speaking with a hushed voice, as if even the word itself is disdainful or unacceptable. We have had the misfortune of meeting some professionals who engage in this type of behaviour, and it demonstrates a significant problem regarding the normalcy of sex, and raises the issue of whether they should be the working with clients who struggle with their sexual behaviour

Conclusion

This book is an important one. The current prevalence of online sex offending behaviour, which continues to grow at an extremely alarming rate, not only within the UK, but globally, indicates that there is something going on that warrants not only further understanding and research, but intervention. The UK criminal justice system takes everything away from these offenders, while society vilifies and ostracises them into isolation, pushing the problem into quarantine like modern day witches or lepers. Therefore, the type of specialist therapeutic work involved with working with this client demographic, including friends, partners and family members, and victims of those currently under investigation, and/or on bail, is not for everyone. It is not unusual during the early stages of therapeutic training for students to be asked whether there are any particular clients or clinical presentations that anyone had specific reservations about working with. Perhaps unsurprisingly, it is 'sex offenders', 'rapists' and 'child molesters' that are most commonly verbalised by many counselling and psychotherapy students. We would argue that surely it is these clients who are potentially struggling the most with connecting themselves to others who would benefit most from someone actively trying to connect and relate to them, and with them. This is why we consider this work is so important, and is fundamentally a child-protection process.

References

Bowlby, J. (1988) *A Secure Base.* Routledge.

Carr, J. (2024) 'There's a crisis going on with men!' YouTube: The Diary of a CEO. https://www.youtube.com/watch?v=uHLAazKUU68.

Christiansen, H.H. (2023) *The exponential growth in data consumption.* LinkedIn. https://www.linkedin.com/pulse/exponential-growth-data-consumption-henrik-h-christiansen-1muuf.

Cooper, A. (2013) *Sex and the Internet. A Guidebook for Clinicians.* Routledge.

Fisher, J. (2021) *Transforming the Living Legacy of Trauma. A Workbook for survivors and therapists.* PESI Publishing.

Golding, K. S. & Hughes, D. A. (2012) *Parenting with PACE to Nurture Confidence and Security in the Troubled Child.* Jessica Kingsley.

Herman, J. L. (1992) *Trauma and Recovery. From domestic abuse to political terror.* Pandora.

Hudson-Allez, G. (2011) *Infant Losses; Adult Searches. A Neural and Developmental Perspective on Psychopathology and Sexual Offending. 2nd Ed.* Karnac.

Hudson-Allez, G. (2023) *A Trauma-Informed Understanding of Online Offending. Adult Losses from Adolescent Searches.* Routledge.

Johnson, R. J., Ross, M. W., Taylor, W. C., Williams, M. L. Carvajal, R. I. & Peters, R. J. (2018) Prevalence of childhood sexual abuse among incarcerated males in county jail. *Child Abuse and Neglect,* 30(1), 75–86.

Jung, C. G. ([1957]2014) *The Undiscovered Self.* Routledge.

Kabat-Zinn, J (2019) *Mindfulness for All. The Wisdom to Transform the World.* Piatkus

Mahmoud, R. (2023) The development of the shadow in childhood and adolescence: Shadow Work: Maia's story. In C. Perry & R. Tower (Eds) *Jung's Shadow Concept. The hidden light and darkness within ourselves.* Routledge.

Maté, G. (2018) *The Realm of Hungry Ghosts: Close Encounters with Addiction.* Vermillion.

Maté, G. & Maté, D. (2024) *The Myth of Normal: Illness, Health and Healing in a Toxic Culture.* Vermillion.

Ogloff, J. R. P., Cutajar, M. C., Mann, E. & Mullen, P. (2012) Child sexual abuse and subsequent offending and victimisation: A follow-up study. *Trends and Issues in Crime and Criminal Justice,* 440, Australian Institute of Criminology. https://www.aic.gov.au/sites/default/files/2020-05/tandi440.pdf.

Panksepp, J. (1998) *Affective Neuroscience. The Foundations of Human and Animal Emotions.* Oxford University Press.

Panksepp, J. & Biven, L. (2021) *The Archaeology of the Mind: neuroevolutionary Origins of Human Emotions.* W.W. Norton & Co.

Porges, S. W. (2017) *The Pocket Guide to the Polyvagal Theory: The Transformative Power of Feeling Safe.* W.W. Norton.

Reicher, S., Haslam, S. A. & Rath, R. (2008) Making a virtue of evil: A five-step social identity model of the development of collective hate. *Social and Personality Psychology Compass,* 2(3), 1313–1344.

Rogers, C. (1977) *On becoming a person. A therapist's view of psychotherapy.* Robinson.

Schore, A. N. (1994) *Affect Regulation and the Origin of the Self. The Neurobiology of Emotional Development.* Lawrence Erlbaum.

Schwartz, M. F., & Southern, S. (2017) Recovery from sexual compulsivity. *Sexual Addiction & Compulsivity: The Journal of Treatment & Prevention,* 24(3), 224–240. doi.org/10.1080/10720162.2017.1350229.

Shapiro, F. (2018) *Eye Movement Desensitization and Reprocessing Therapy (EMDR) Basic Principles, Protocols and Procedures. 3rd ed.* Guilford Press.

Chapter 2

The victim's voice

Antounette Philippides

Introduction

Conducting therapeutic interventions with victims of sexual abuse as well as with perpetrators aids therapists in achieving a helpful balance and insight into all aspects of the offending behaviour, which informs the therapy, and encourages a unique richness to the work. In this chapter, I will explore victim presentations in therapy to demonstrate that there is often an embodiment of deep complex feelings and how, with the guidance and support of a therapist, the individual can emotionally grow to take control and become a survivor of the abuse. This process, described to me by a survivor client, is a transitional process, which is necessary for the both the health and the wellbeing of the individual. In writing this, I have used the term 'victim' in the title as opposed to 'survivor', because this reflects the situation that many partners, survivors of abuse and other family members of perpetrators, present at the start of therapy.

Often, the initial stages of therapy with those affected by the abusive actions of perpetrators are full of mixed emotions that can be confusing, life-changing and too often, life-limiting. Therapy with a victim is a complex process that merits exploration, because we may not always be able to prevent the first crime, but ensuring the abused person is treated with respect, care, kindness and compassion will go a long way to heal the hurt caused. Anger, grief, shame, embarrassment, denial and many other 'heavy weight' emotions all loom large in the therapy room. They all need to be given oxygen in the therapy to enable the person before us to process their own situation; to seek as much acceptance as they can or want in order to live the best life they can going forward. What therapy cannot do is undo the wrongs of the past. This is a difficult concept to come to terms with as clients and practitioners. As trauma-informed therapists, how many of us would love to achieve that level of healing?

Who are the victims that come to StopSO for therapy?

StopSO offers therapy to any and all victims and survivors of abuse. Mostly, they are adults who present as victims from their childhood, who have reached the point

DOI: 10.4324/9781003509103-3

of needing specialist intervention. Somehow, their experience of abuse has surfaced and is interrupting their progress, or they are plagued by memories, flashbacks, thoughts and emotions of fear, panic or anger, or all three. Their experience has now become an impediment to their growth as an individual and within their relationships. All of these feelings need to be acknowledged and worked through within the therapy. There are a number of 'types' of relationship to the perpetrator that have culminated in people feeling they are victims of their behaviour. There are three typical types of victims: those who were directly abused, either recently or historically, in childhood or in adulthood; there are the partners of an individual accused or convicted of a sexual offence and/or their children, often described as secondary victims, (see Chapters 3 and 8); and there are perpetrators who were victims themselves historically who have become abusers. In this chapter we will address each type of victim presentation and offer a case study to highlight the work involved.

Victims who were physically, sexually or emotionally abused

The greatest damage to an individual is often conducted during childhood when traumatic experiences of domestic violence or sexual violation occur and damage a developing child's brain, most notably occurring when the child's sexual template comes online between the ages of six and nine years (Hudson-Allez, 2011). Neglect in early years can equally have a devastating effect on the emotional and psychological development of the person (Stauffer, 2021). It is considered that the deepest wound inflicted on a child occurs when the abuser is a parent, creating a conflict between the person who is supposed to love you the most and the person who hurts you the most (van der Kolk, 2015).

'Adele'

Adele, a 25-year-old woman, in work, living with parents. She attends therapy because she drinks too much, takes recreational drugs at the weekend and has no idea why she feels compelled to do either of these things to excess regularly. It impacts on her ability to focus at work, her relationships, her finances and her mood is concerningly low.

Therapy is her 'last resort'; she cannot drink her way out of feeling 'pointless'. After therapy had begun, she mentioned, quite low key, that she hated family gatherings. Then she let rip. Boy did she hate family gatherings! Her step brother, 18 months older, would use these opportunities to abuse her, from the age of 11 until she was 17. Every time the family got together, he *would target her. As this persisted, her self-worth plummeted, although it was not apparent to her until, in therapy, she revealed for the first time why family gatherings were so abhorrent to her.*

This young lady did not realise she was a victim as she did not identify her step-brother's behaviour as abuse, nor did she connect her addiction to what therapists would identify as trauma. Therapeutic work supported her in these realisations. Gabor Maté argued, 'When it comes to understanding addiction, the dilemma of not seeing is deep. Our defences will not allow us to be aware of our own pain and the dysfunctions in which we seek escape from it' (Maté, 2018, p. 24). The therapy needs to give the client time to come to terms with this realisation, which may mean reframing her understanding of her whole life. Then, when she is ready, to help her to manage her reactions to the events, which she manifested in alcohol addiction, enabling her to stay in the here and now, and not to dissociate from herself in order to cope with the emotional and physical pain of the past.

Here are some common **psychological** reactions to trauma:

- Losing hope for the future (hopelessness)
- Feeling distant (detached) or losing a sense of concern about others (dissociation)
- Being unable to concentrate or make decisions
- Feeling jumpy and getting startled easily at sudden noises
- Feeling on guard and alert all the time (hypervigilance)
- Having upsetting dreams and memories (flashbacks)
- Having problems at work or school
- Avoiding people, places and things related to the event

They may also experience more **physical** reactions such as:

- Stomach upset and trouble eating
- Trouble sleeping and feeling very tired
- Pounding heart, rapid breathing, feeling shaky
- Sweating
- Severe headache if thinking of the event
- Not keeping up with exercise, diet, safe sex or regular health care
- Smoking more, using alcohol or drugs more or eating too much
- Having ongoing medical problems get worse

They may have **emotional** troubles such as:

- Feeling nervous, helpless, fearful, sad
- Feeling shocked, numb, or not able to feel love or joy

- Being irritable or having angry outbursts
- Getting easily upset or agitated
- Blaming themselves or having negative views of themselves or the world
- Being unable to trust others, getting into fights, or trying to control everything
- Being withdrawn, feeling rejected, or abandoned
- Feeling detached, not wanting intimacy

(National Centre for PTSD, 2024)

Judith Lewis Herman maintained that these distress symptoms described above simultaneously called attention to the existence of the 'unspeakable secret' of trauma, whilst also deflecting attention from it (Herman, 2001). Therefore, working with this duality is the substance of the therapeutic work, which helps the client's understanding of the impact of trauma they experienced. Therapy helps the client revisit their pain, and remove any secrecy, but also provides some psychoeducation to normalise what is happening to them, so that they can manage, with delicacy, the pain and damage that abuse causes.

Non-offending partners of perpetrators (NOP)

StopSO works with partners or wives of perpetrators of (mostly) men, who are under investigation for viewing, making and/or distributing child sexual abuse material (CSAM). Increasingly, the charges they face are also reflecting the Artificial Intelligence (AI) world and since Covid, grooming charges from online chat rooms which have escalated (Skidmore, Aitkenhead & Muir, 2022). Women and men in relationships with men who have committed these crimes have a complex set of emotions to understand and explore. When 'the knock' comes, the NOPs are plunged into the world of pornography use and criminal behaviours of their partners/husbands, and are made brutally aware of their partner's sexual activity outside of them.

'Brenda'

Brenda is a 28-year-old woman nursing her five-week-old baby. The police have removed her husband's devices and have taken him to the police station. No-one tells her why. Her thoughts as to why and what he may have done become increasingly fantastical. But at no point does she consider he has been viewing illegal images of children, or that he had been indulging in a pornography compulsion. That information was not made clear to her until he returned to their home to collect his belongings to reside elsewhere. As with so many partners, she is forcibly plunged into becoming aware of the world of pornography and of child abuse. She had believed that he had been 'the perfect partner': a caring, attentive, sensitive husband. She could have wanted for no more. She attended for therapy four months later still in a state of shock and disbelief.

Here, the therapeutic work needs to focus on her coming to terms with accepting the painful reality that he was not perfect. He was hiding a secret, the exposure of which would change the course of her life. The issue of secondary trauma and how to work with it is addressed in Chapter 8. However, for this case, I was aware that she lost her sense of self the day the police attended, and needed to grieve the loss of all she had believed to be her truth. As a therapist, balancing the palpable pain of a partner such as Brenda's with the next session of the day, who may be a perpetrator focusing on identifying his needs, can be challenging. This is where the need for good supervision and support is paramount.

Victims of historical abuse who have become abusers

There is a perspective that it is a myth that those who were abused will become abusers, or have a greater chance of become a perpetrator. However, we can never *really* know how many people were abused and did not become abusers. Seeking statistical analysis of how many perpetrators were abused, it seems, is only part of the story of the impact of abuse. However, research suggests 35% of perpetrators had reported childhood sexual abuse experiences, often by a female relative (Glasser et al., 2001). Equally however, parental loss in childhood was also a strong predictor of a trajectory between victim to perpetrator. This suggests it is not just abuse that leads people to sexually harm others, but traumatic life events that can be a predisposing factor (Hudson-Allez, 2023).

StopSO accepts that perpetrators of sexual abuse may have a history of abuse. In fact, in contrast to some other agencies working in this field, we embrace perpetrators who fully engage therapeutically who wish to discuss their history of abuse, as they will often have the goal of wanting to understand why they had committed the offence. I cannot condone an organisational approach that makes therapeutic support available to survivors and yet rejects these same clients at the point of disclosure of an offence. The potential impact of this is to cause the client, who embodies the dual position of victim and perpetrator, to condemnation for their offending without due care and attention to their own trauma.

As a society, we condemn perpetrators. They have caused harm to the most vulnerable in our communities. The need for punishment looms large in a collective psyche that feels justified in inhabiting the echo chamber encouraged by social media and the media in general. Headlines that labels and dehumanises perpetrators as 'monsters', or worse, do not allow or consider a different perspective encouraged by good therapy, asking not 'what have you done?' but 'what happened to you?'.

This is not a monochrome world we inhabit. The bad people versus the innocent is not a space that therapy can inhabit. Therapy reaches the part of clients that is in pain and discomfort and looks at the shadow side of themselves. If this has manifested in their abuse of others, then this is what the therapy must focus upon. If there is a history of trauma, as so often there is, then we work with this. In the cases I am considering, the trauma is abuse, and the manifestation is abuse. Rejecting the client for perpetrating abuse will not support him/her to desist, to understand and to heal.

'Charles'

Charles is a 42-year-old man who is struggling to stop viewing child sexual abuse material (CSAM). He was arrested a year ago and after a six-month investigation was released NFA (No Further Action). He had returned to the family home where he lived with his wife and two children under ten years of age. He started therapy and after debriefing his current circumstances and reporting a developmental history, he told the therapist, 'I don't know what happened in my childhood, but I recall his [father's] hands all over my body in the night'. The details of his abuse had become buried behind a dissociative amnestic barrier. The work, slowly and with equal measures of pain and healing, unpicked his experience and the legacy of the abuse. This provided the road to his recovery, from his perceived need to explore CSAM to a position of self-acceptance that he was a victim of his father's actions; but that he can survive this and allow himself to be the best version of himself he can. His own abuse had placed a glass ceiling on his willingness to engage his 'free child' in any aspect of his life. As a therapist, being party to the release of such an innate right to joy is a privilege.

I am delighted that StopSO will embrace the work with survivors when they are also perpetrators. I have considered the perspective that those who have been abused cannot 'recover' as the damage done cannot be undone. This I regard as short-sighted and frankly offensive. Such an attitude condemns victims to living a life with limitation. 'Where brutal interactions do occur, they are thought to be the cause of **trauma**: a potentially irreparable injury to the person's psyche, and a potential cause of mental disorders' (Middleton, Sachs & Dorahy, 2017, p. 249). This should not be not the perspective of a therapist. We seek to journey to healing and acceptance.

The relationship between the abuser and the victim can be very complex. I am considering the relationship of a child victim attending therapy as an adult, whose perpetrator was a family, trusted friend or relative. It is emotive, shrouded in a secrecy that, however uncomfortable, binds the survivor to the perpetrator. Secrets and silence were the cornerstone of maintaining the sense of 'specialness' for the victim. Accepting the damage caused requires an awareness of the wrongness of the relationship. Clients passage through grief at this point; letting go of what as a child was a time of attention and 'specialness', and acknowledging the pain (somatic, emotional and psychological) can be difficult but necessary. It can be present in therapy as a survivor minimising the abuse they suffered. Disentangling the relationship from the harm done through the relationship is as painful as the harm itself.

'Donald'

Donald was a 52-year-old male, who was sexually abused by a family friend that his dad entrusted him to after his mum died and dad had to work. He was seven years of age. He described the abuse as 'gentle, caring, never caused me physical harm. It was not brutal, like rape'. When he was 19, a friend of similar age, raped him; this was forced and brutal, needing medical intervention. No-one in authority, in education, in his family or at his work asked why he was 'a bit odd', or 'acted badly or disobediently'. He had few friends and struggled to communicate his feelings. When his friend (rapist) came to see him subsequent to the rape, there was a fight and Donald launched into what the Crown Prosecution Service described as an 'unprovoked brutal attack on a visiting friend'. He was sentenced to two years custody. Therapy considered these complex relationships in detail. It enabled and encouraged Donald to give voice to his feelings. However, any consideration of the relationship with his original abuser was initially shrouded in the gentleness with which he felt he had physically penetrated him. There was certainly a cruelty to the realisation that this too was a brutality of immense proportions.

It used to be considered that any consideration regarding an offender's own traumatic background should be discussed later rather than in the early stages of treatment; that while 'the abuser is still deep into his own feelings about himself his thinking about the abuse he has committed is distorted, so that he justifies and minimises it rather than genuinely attempting to empathise with his victim/s' (Renvoize, 1993, p.107). However, when one revisits the list of physical, emotional and psychological presentations described above, it becomes clear that the therapist *must* deal with this historical trauma *first*, in order to make space for the person to think about others, free from the constant hypervigilance, dissociation and rumination of past injustices. This needs to be conducted slowly and delicately. Babette Rothschild likened the process to one of a pressure cooker that needs to be released slowly and safely a little at a time. If the client is opened up too quickly, the pressure becomes extreme and can lead to an explosion: decompensation, breakdown, serious illness or suicide (Rothschild, 2000). She argues for the judicious use of 'the brakes' so that the whole process of trauma therapy becomes less risky.

So we ask the same question in different ways; we ask: 'what happened to you?'. It is the exploration of this, with perpetrators as well as victims, that enables the individual to understand better; for victims to place blame away from themselves, and for perpetrators to accept that very same blame. With all clients, managing that blame and shame is a significant step forward in their lives.

Conclusion

Working therapeutically with clients who have been victimised is complex, and needs a compassionate and caring way of being, whether they are victims of physical, sexual or emotional abuse; whether they are victimised by proxy by society and by the State as a consequence of the offence committed by a husband or partner; or whether the victim turns abuser, as in the minority of cases. All deserve our non-judgemental, authentic support over what tends to be long and delicate therapeutic work.

References

Glasser, M., Kolvin, I., Campbell, D. Glasser, A & Farrelly, S. (2001) Cycle of child sexual abuse: Links between being a victim and becoming a perpetrator. *British Journal of Psychiatry,* 179, 482–494.

Herman J. L. (2001) *Trauma and Recovery. From Domestic Abuse to Political Terror.* Pandora.

Hudson-Allez, G. (2011) *Infant Losses; Adult Searches. A Neural and Developmental Perspective on Psychopathology and Sexual Offending. 2nd ed.* Karnac.

Hudson-Allez, G. (2023) *A Trauma-Informed Understanding of Online Offending. Adult Losses from Adolescent Searches.* Routledge.

Maté, G. (2018) *In the Realm of Hungry Ghosts: Close Encounters with Addiction.* Vermillion.

Middleton, W., Sachs, A. & Dorahy, M. J. (2017) The abused and the abuser: Victim-perpetrator dynamics. *Journal of Trauma Dissociation,* 18(3), 249–258. DOI:10.1080/15 299732.2017.1295373.

National Centre for PTSD (2024) https://www.ptsd.va.gov/index.asp.

Renvoize, J. (1993) *Innocence Destroyed. A Study of Child Sexual Abuse.* Routledge.

Rothschilds, B. (2000) *The Body Remembers. The Psychophysiology of Trauma and Trauma Treatment.* Norton.

Skidmore, M., Aitkenhead, B. & Muir, R. (2022) *Turning the Tide Against Online Child Sexual Abuse.* The Police Foundation.

Stauffer, K. A. (2021). *Emotional neglect and the adult in therapy.* Norton.

van der Kolk, B. (2015) *The Body keeps the Score: Brain, Mind and Body Healing of Trauma.* Penguin.

Chapter 3

Addressing trauma and secondary harms in families where a parent is suspected of possession of child sexual abuse material

Michael Sheath

UK police arrest around 850 suspects per month for offences relating to the possession of child sexual exploitation material (Centre of Expertise, 2023). Around half of these suspects will be living in a household with children, and the majority of those individuals will be the father of those children. The early morning arrival of police officers executing a warrant, colloquially referred to as 'the knock', triggers a significant degree of stress and trauma in families, with the suspect being at significant risk of suicide as a result of his arrest, partners being at very high risk of experiencing post-traumatic stress (PTSD) symptoms, and children being confused and stigmatised. Criminal investigations into the possession and distribution of child sexual exploitation material are both necessary and inevitable; this chapter will not argue otherwise. However, what were once unintended and unforeseen negative consequences of those investigations are now well documented and foreseeable. In the light of that, a more sophisticated and nuanced response needs to be adopted by law enforcement and children's services.

Primary and secondary harms

Primary harms will not be directly addressed in this chapter, but they will influence the discourse. They include the possibility that the suspect has been sexually abusing children in the household or elsewhere, and that his conduct is indicative of his harbouring a sexual interest in, or sexual ambition towards, children. These direct and prospective dangers posed to children by viewers of CSAM will be considered elsewhere in this book. Suffice it to say here that a vigorous and evolving debate persists as to the crossover between what might colloquially be referred to as 'viewing' and 'doing'. Secondary harms refer to the unintended consequences of the criminal investigation and the revelation of the suspect's conduct, be that his suicide, his partner's trauma, the family's disintegration and so on. The secondary harms referred to in this chapter are universal, and are not necessarily increased or reduced by the direct risk posed by the suspect. Nor, it seems, are secondary harms reduced by the decisions a partner might make: divorce, 'standing by' the suspect, allowing contact or resisting contact, do not appear to have a substantial impact in amplifying or reducing secondary harms.

DOI: 10.4324/9781003509103-4

The trigger for the trauma seems to be located in two events: the revelation of the suspect's conduct, and how the family manages it whilst subject to state scrutiny. The state, through its agencies, needs to tread carefully when it involves itself in family life.

Iatrogenic harm

Historic examples of secondary harm are worth considering. The most poignant relates to the work of a Hungarian physician, Ignaz Semmelweiss, who worked and studied in a maternity clinic in Vienna in the 1840s (Semmelweiss, 1858). He noted that the maternal death rate in one clinic was consistently double that of another in the same location. In one year, 16% of the women giving birth died of puerperal fever. The 'safer' clinic was staffed by student midwives, the other by student doctors. It transpired that the student doctors would migrate from dissecting corpses as part of their studies to assisting with births without washing their hands between locations; the midwives had only one task and on that basis cross-contamination did not feature. Semmelweiss, against some resistance, initiated a strict regime of hand washing that reduced the death rate to 1%. In writing up his work for academic journals, Semmelweiss was widely criticised and derided by the medical establishment, and died at the hands of wardens in a mental asylum after having suffered a breakdown. The concept of iatrogenic harm, essentially 'harms caused by doctors' is worth considering as analogous to the secondary harms considered in this chapter. Well-intentioned and professional, police and children's services practitioners have occasionally and inadvertently generated one set of harms whilst legitimately trying to avert others.

Primary, secondary and tertiary prevention

Notions of prevention have been in the ascendancy in work related to the sexual exploitation of children for some decades now, with Smallbone, Marshall and Wortley's (2013) Public Health model gaining substantial traction. Smallbone, Marshall and Wortley suggested the sexual exploitation of children might best be regarded as a disease, akin to malaria or diabetes, and that long-standing public health improvement strategies might be employed as a means of reducing or eradicating it. In this model, *primary prevention* strategies relate to universal messages that might be offered to the public: 'don't smoke', 'drink less alcohol', 'get vaccinated'. In the case of sexual exploitation, these interventions might relate to raising awareness, challenging taboos, offering advice, challenging rape myths and so forth. *Secondary prevention* targets those at greater risk, such as where general practitioners (GPs) might screen patients who present at greater risk of a heart attack because of their lifestyle. In a sexual exploitation reduction strategy, one might engage men on pornography sites whose search terms indicate they may be shifting towards abusive or violent content. *Tertiary prevention* seeks to deal with the consequences of a medical episode: the stroke victim is hospitalised and rehabilitated, the man who sexually abuses a child is reported, arrested, tried and convicted, and receives counselling in prison; the sexually abused child is given therapy, and so on. In all cases where tertiary prevention strategies are applied, the damage has already been done, notions of 'moving upstream' to primary and secondary prevention strategies have become central to the current prevention discourse.

What is missing from Smallbone and Wortley's offering is the notion of *quaternary prevention*, or 'action taken to protect individuals from medical interventions that are likely to cause more harm than good' (Martins, Godycki-Cwirko & Heleno, 2018, p. 1). This takes us back to Semmelweiss's interventions in Vienna. In respect to sexual exploitation reduction, the system ought to provide advice and campaigns that are realistic and not victim-blaming, shifting responsibility from children to 'keep themselves safe' to focus on adult perpetrators and prospective perpetrators, avoiding campaigns based upon unrealistic and unhelpful notions of 'stranger danger', ensuring that systems for managing child witnesses reduce rather than amplify their trauma, and so forth (Harris, Sheath & Shields, 2024). The rest of this chapter considers the iatrogenic harms caused by, or connected to, necessary police investigations into the viewing and sharing of child sexual abuse material, referred to as CSAM from this point.

Consequences of policing and prosecution

It is important to contextualise the policing and prosecution of individuals involved in viewing and collecting, and sometimes disseminating CSAM. All are involved in viewing images that depict or promote the sexual abuse of children, and they are connected to the child's ongoing victimisation. In the earliest sentencing guidelines from the turn of the millennium, they are described as being 'complicit in the original abuse of the child' (Sentencing Council for England and Wales, 2002) and it is clear that the individual viewing images generates further trauma for those so depicted. Beyond those certainties, matters become more complex. Some viewers will have a history of direct abuse of children, whether it has been discovered or not. Many viewers will not have a history of direct abuse, but they *may* be on a trajectory that leads to escalation. The difficulty for the police, and for children's services, and indeed for the partners of these men, is that at the point of their arrest these issues will be unresolved. The challenge for the authorities, in the interim, is to safeguard the children in the household, but society needs to be more specific and explicit about the meaning of safeguarding in these contexts. Safeguarding is not simply achieved by removing the suspect from the household, but includes minimising and ameliorating the negative consequences that flow from 'the knock' itself.

Trauma has been defined as 'any disturbing experience that results in significant fear, helplessness, dissociation, confusion and other disruptive feelings intense enough to have a long-lasting negative effect on a person's attitudes, behaviour, and other aspects of functioning' (APA, 2018). By that definition, 'the knock' qualifies: involving an early morning visit by police officers to a household where, typically, the viewer of indecent material is the only member of the household who immediately knows why the police are present. Adult men are overwhelmingly the suspect, although in very recent years it transpires that adolescent boys feature as significant consumers of abusive content (Grant, 2023). In the main, it is the wife or partner of the offender and the mother of his children who has to manage the revelation.

As early as 2015, Stubley noted two main psychological struggles engaged in by women whose partner had been arrested for possession of CSAM (Stubley, 2015). One was the initial shock of discovery, which Stubley describes as 'stunned blindsidedness', with her suggesting the consequences of the arrest were so severe that they removed the woman's capacity to function, a description that was later validated by the work of Armitage and The Lucy Faithfull Foundation (Armitage et al., 2023). It is important to realise that it is not uncommon, on the same day as the partner is arrested, for the non-offending partner to be visited by Children's Services' workers and asked about their attitude to the alleged offending. Ambivalence, denial, minimisation and simple incoherence might be taken as evidence of an inability to protect, or collusiveness, when in fact they are better regarded as an archetypal and indicative of a traumatic experience. The second struggle for women in these situations is in the longer term: managing the children, deciding who within the circle of family and friends might be informed, and who might be supportive, dealing with 'the authorities' and their expectations, and making life-changing decisions about contact, divorce, reconciliation and support at a time when no certainty can be found. This second phase can last for any period from eighteen months to five years or longer, depending on how the criminal matter might be resolved and how any public or private law proceedings might evolve. The extinguishing of contact between a father and his children may appear to provide a solution to anxieties about the children's welfare, but it may also create enormous difficulties for the child in terms of guilt and divided loyalties. In any event, the conviction of a father for what is essentially a sexual offence is, regardless of any criminal or civil outcome, is likely to have a profound impact on the children's sense of identity.

The sudden and usually unexpected discovery that a partner has been viewing images of children being sexually abused has regularly been described as 'like a death' (Sheath, 2022). This was expressed directly to me during the course of my own work conducting assessments into women's 'ability to protect' for the Family Courts from 1997 until 2022. The experience parallels Colin Murray Parkes' (Parkes, 2009) work on bereavement, and this realisation was explicitly reflected in a joint Barnardo's and Stop it Now! Scotland report published in 2016 (Families Outside, 2016). Most readers will be familiar with the experience of bereavement:

- *Disbelief* being archetypal: the dead person cannot have left us and is willed to return.
- *Anger* at the medical services involved who ought to have saved them, or at the person themselves for leading an unhealthy lifestyle.

- *Bargaining*, or 'trying to make it good', with appeals to God or promises to be a better person will always be futile and any prayers will be unanswered.
- *Sadness*, possibly depression, in most cases.
- *Acceptance* of the reality of death following.

Women faced with the suggestion that their partner has been involved in criminal and sexually deviant conduct will typically deny it. Cognitive dissonance exists where a previous view of a partner as a good father and good partner (although there are exceptions to this) is challenged by the suggestion that he is 'a paedophile' or 'a sex criminal', and an initial rejection of that is to be expected rather than regarded as evidence of a failure to protect. Women may express anger at the police or Children's Services for intruding into their family life, or even at themselves for 'failing' to notice their partner's hidden behaviour. Bargaining might be expressed in terms of guilt, that if they had been more engaged, more loving or more competent at meeting their partner's needs, then he may not have strayed; a myth that some men may utilise as a means of defraying blame in any event. Sadness and resignation may follow, since the family can never be the same after 'the knock', regardless of any practical outcome. Acceptance may never come.

Core assumptions

Other theories assist in understanding the dilemmas and traumas that non-offending partners in these situations experience, and I have made it a habit, in practice, to share them with clients rather than simply write about them to referrers. Shattered Assumptions Theory (Janoff-Bulman, 1992) is based upon notions of schema, which are essentially assumptions that usually help us to navigate the social world. Janoff-Bulman suggested that individuals will experience a state of high anxiety and fear if and when their schema or core assumptions about the world are challenged by an unexpected and unwanted experience. In many cases where a family is engaged by what must appear to be the terrifying arm of the state, that family will have had very little prior experience of the authorities. The vast majority of men arrested for possession of CSAM have no previous convictions for instance. A woman's settled view, that the world is a benevolent, predictable and ordered place, and that since she is good, no evil will come to her will be challenged by the early morning arrival of police officers, however sympathetic their approach, and by her own and her children's security being placed at risk; be that by her partner or (in her view) by the authorities themselves. This sense, that what seemed previously ordered, just and predictable is suddenly chaotic, unfair and unpredictable presents a significant challenge, with anger, denial, impotence and depression being perfectly predictable and reasonable responses to it. One of the ironies of the experience of 'the knock' is that most women subjected to it will have had a reasonably ordered life experience, free of trauma, until that point; this leaves them especially vulnerable to experiencing trauma.

Trauma for the non-offending partner

Armitage's research on trauma (Armitage, 2023) was based upon interviews with women who had contacted the Stop it Now! Helpline after their partner had been arrested. One issue that emerged was the discovery of remarkably high levels of Post-Traumatic Stress Disorder (PTSD) in the cohort of women who engaged with researchers and completed the Impact of Events Scale-R (Weiss & Marmar, 1997), which is a self-report measure designed to measure traumatic stress symptoms. A score of between 24 and 33 would be clinically concerning, a score over 34 would be deemed indicative of PTSD, and a score over 37 would be associated with a suppression of immune system functioning and thereby create physical symptoms and ill health. Of the 45 respondents, 70% scored over 34, with 65% scoring over 37, meaning their immune system was likely to be compromised.

It is important to note here that during this same period the woman would be required to look after their children, manage issues relating to the relationship with their partner and its continuance or extinction and offer a coherent, insightful and protective view of matters to the authorities. There appeared to be no meaningful difference, in terms of trauma symptoms, between women who ended their relationship with their partner and those who chose to continue with it in conditions they described as 'strained'. The exception to high levels of trauma symptomology was where the woman continued with the relationship and felt it was 'stronger'; one might speculate that the couple clung together in opposition to a common enemy, or that the revelation of the partner's offending caused him, or them, to re-evaluate how the relationship might be conducted.

Armitage also considered (Armitage et al., 2022) common experiences or themes described by the women she and her researchers engaged. Seven themes emerged:

1. *Disenfranchised grief* connects with notions of bereavement, although in this case the loss of a partner cannot be discussed as it might be as if he had died. Bystanders withhold support, or make it conditional upon the woman taking a certain stance she might not, in her heart, support. Feelings of loss might be denied or minimised, misunderstood or misrepresented. The usual offerings of empathy and sympathy are suspended.
2. *Ambiguous loss* refers to '*a loss that is unclear, unverified, often without resolution*'. Unlike death, the loss of a partner, or the threat of it, cannot be resolved; there can be no permanence or resolution to it, and a stigma may attach to the woman who grieves, since some onlookers may feel she is wrong to mourn the loss of some kind of monster.
3. *Ontological assault* connects to the nature of the woman's identity: who is she after 'the knock'? Her role as a wife may be extinguished, her role as a mother is subject to the judgement of professional others, her identity as a woman may be challenged by simple gossip: 'What sort of woman can be married to a man like that?' Image, reputation, and identity are all challenged, including by the

woman herself: 'Who am I?' 'Who was he?' may be common questions, attached to self-blame that she had 'failed' to notice anything awry, or if she had, that she had failed to act.

4. *Contamination by causal responsibility* encapsulates the charge that she 'should have known, or must have known' about her partner's criminality, or that a 'better' woman would have acted in such a way as to prevent a man's straying sexuality.

5. *Wall of silence* which may be created by the suspect himself, with him refusing to discuss or explain his conduct, potentially through shame and anxiety or possibly through a form of emotional control and coercion. He may seek to control the narrative, blaming his viewing CSAM as being the result of a computer virus or upon stress, or pornography addiction, which may in truth be valid but is almost inevitably offered as a sole cause. The couple may agree a false narrative to placate their friends and neighbours and as a means of explaining the suspect's absence from the home. The authorities themselves may keep the partner in ignorance of what they suspect, through reference to Data Protection principles, or as a means of securing evidence.

6. *A rock and a hard place*: women frequently describe being criticised if they support their partner, or condemned if they do not.

7. *A burden of responsibility* is invariably placed upon women who, as described above, are frequently traumatised in their own right. Despite that, they are viewed as the principal agent of protection or 'protective factor' in the case, and will be expected to manage and supervise contact, keep the children informed and consoled and support their partner if he is at risk of suicide.

In many ways, the traumatic experience of women in these situations mirrors that of direct victims of child sexual abuse. Finkelhor's (1986) exploration of what he termed *traumagenic dynamics* can be adapted to explore the forces at work when a partner is under investigation for a form of vicarious child sexual exploitation. Four elements are considered:

- **Sexualisation** refers to the engagement of a child in activities that they are not psychologically, culturally or physically prepared for: the notion of an 'age of consent' in almost all cultures reinforces a perspective that premature sexual experiences are intrinsically harmful. The additional notion here is that it is the psychological impact of abuse that is as potent as the physical harms. A sexually abused child may grow to associate sex with pain, humiliation, fear, punishment or reward. The consequences may be an adult life blighted by anxiety, confusion, arousal problems and sexual dysfunction. Adult women dealing with the consequences of their partner's downloading face traumatic and intrusive thoughts: was their partner abusing their children? Was he thinking about the images of children when he was intimate with her? What is the truth of his sexuality? Some women experience the revelation as being akin to the discovery of infidelity, where the object of desire is not another woman, but a child.

- **Stigma** attaches to children who are sexually abused, with perpetrators using blame and misdirection to make the child feel responsible for their own abuse, creating feelings of shame and guilt where none ought to exist. Bystanders frequently question children's motives for disclosing, or for 'failing' to disclose, or opine that teenage victims of sexual exploitation might have 'protected themselves' or 'made better choices'. Partners of men found to have been viewing CSAM might be regarded with suspicion; their blamelessness is doubted. If they support their partner they are seen as collusive; if they reject him, they are seen as disloyal. They might be seen as bad wives, bad mothers and bad women.
- **Betrayal.** A sense of betrayal attaches to children who are sexually abused, since in most cases the perpetrator is someone they and their family know and trust; familiarity is the greatest ally of the groomer. It is unsurprising, thereafter, that a child may be sceptical about the good intentions of others, including professionals. Women subject to 'the knock' are likely to feel an acute sense of betrayal at the partner's conduct, and at his putting them at risk of the scrutiny and judgement of both the state and of neighbours, family and friends. Anger at the partner, disappointment at his conduct and anxiety as to how matters might be resolved are likely to become crippling; a lack of trust in the authorities attempting to resolve matters is to be expected, rather than being viewed as a failure to engage.
- **Powerlessness** attaches to an experience of sexual abuse, since the child is engaged in sexual and intimate activities against their will and interests. Children abused in secrecy and shame may adopt the point of view of their abuser, and believe his suggestion that he was led on by them, could not resist them, was acting out of love, or that they 'deserved it' in some way. This experience amplifies the child's sense impotence, challenges any ambition to self-determination, and produces depression, fatalism and lower self-esteem. Women under scrutiny by the state and neighbourhood after the arrest of their partner face two challenges: one is that their partner may lie, or obfuscate about the true nature of his behaviour and his motivation for it; the power of that knowledge rests with him. Secondly she has to deal with necessary enquiries as to her children's safety. If she rejects the notion of her partner's prospective or assumed dangerousness, she is likely to be regarded as unprotective. If she accepts it, she may be suspected of what is termed 'disguised compliance' if disbelieved, or services might be withdrawn if she is believed since she will be regarded as representing 'a protective factor', thus absolving the state of any further need to engage.

Damage to children

The goal of state intervention in these cases is simply referred to as safeguarding. The assumption is, typically, that the resident father poses a direct sexual risk to the children, and given that, the intervention is designed to minimise or extinguish risk.

As mentioned above, these primary dangers are usually the only dangers contemplated, and they ought not be minimised. Some fathers do create CSAM involving their own children, and some fathers consume CSAM as part of a wider range of behaviours which might include the online engagement of children. At the point of 'the knock' these matters are usually moot, and in many cases, they remain unresolved. The parents may separate as a result of the stress the family is subject to, and a compromise over contact between the father and children may be negotiated outside the scrutiny of the Family Courts.

Wider notions of the children's wellbeing as it is affected prior to and during their father being subject to a criminal enquiry might usefully be addressed through the lens of the Adverse Childhood Experiences (ACE) study (Centre for Disease Control, 1998.) This considers ten negative childhood experiences, and suggests that in combination, a conglomeration of these experiences produces increasing negative adult outcomes, affecting physical and mental health and, ultimately, the prospect of an early death. The simple underpinning of the study is the understanding that children subject to abuses, neglects and stresses experience such levels of stress that their brain development is interfered with, and they develop means of managing trauma that are themselves damaging to health. The actuarial tables in relation to high ACE scores make for arresting reading. A child who enters adulthood with an ACE score over six has a 30-fold risk of suicide than an average child, with a seven-fold risk of developing a dependence upon alcohol with a score over four. These are, of course, average risk factors, and not immutable or determinative, but they do offer a call to action that childhood traumas need to be reduced. In any event, at its core, the ACE study suggests a society is well advised to minimise the abuse, trauma and neglect of its children since the impacts of it are both lifelong and life reducing.

One can consider the elements of the ACE scale in two contexts: one is the possible harms caused to children during the course of their father's criminal conduct, when it is undiscovered. The other is the possible harms caused or resulting from the revelation and investigation of their father's criminal conduct. Nothing mentioned here suggests that investigations into such matters ought not be conducted. The implications are more that thought ought to given to managing and minimising secondary harms, because they can be foreseen.

Seven of the ten elements of the ACE scale are considered here: *Physical abuse*, *Physical neglect* and *Mother treated violently* are not typically present in households occupied by a downloader of CSAM, although care needs be taken since these experiences are archetypally secret and denied, particularly domestic violence. One can, however, be more confident of the likely presence of other harms. *Sexual abuse* must, of course, be considered as a possibility in any household occupied by someone viewing CSAM. Since children are more likely to be sexually abused by a family member than a stranger, and identified victims of CSAM production are most likely to be found living in the same household as the abuser, initial caution in taking a view of the father is warranted. The difficulty is that in most investigations, this is the only issue considered; harms resulting from the involvement of the state are not considered on a routine basis by the majority of police forces and by almost no children's services' departments.

Emotional abuse may be experienced by children living in proximity to a CSAM viewer since he may hold negative or abusive views of children in general, or be in thrall to sites hosting incest content. Those attitudes may leak into his engagement with his own offspring. After his conduct becomes known to others, particularly by way of social media, the children may be subject to abusive comment by their peers. *Emotional neglect* may feature in children's lives because one parent is preoccupied with indecent online content, and has neither the time nor the inclination to engage with his children.

Once 'the knock' has been experienced, children will be parented by one or both parents who are themselves likely to be traumatised, and may lack the emotional energy to manage their children's distress too. In most cases, at least in the short to medium term, it is the mother who is called upon to protect and comfort the children, and explain something she may be barely able to understand and manage herself. *Household substance abuse* creates stress in family life, and various neglects and pressures. It is not uncommon, in my experience, to find that a man who has been repeatedly visiting CSAM sites has other compelling habits: alcohol and stimulant drugs such as cocaine and amphetamines are frequently cited as accompanying and occasionally complementing periods of downloading. Inevitably, some individuals will manage trauma by resorting to intoxicants; this may create an adverse experience for children that was not in train beforehand. *Household mental illness* might be present, prior to a disclosure, because some downloaders embark upon an episode of CSAM viewing as part of a wider experience of dysphoria. Post-disclosure, it is common to find one or both parents in a depressed and anxious state that renders normal parenting impossible. This connects with suicide, which is not regarded as an ACE, but which common sense and simple empathy would indicate offers a profound challenge to children's well-being.

Incarcerated family member is the penultimate ACE considered here, which together with *Parental separation or divorce* are the two 'post hoc' consequences of discovered downloading that may affect children. The impacts of parental imprisonment, including absence and stigma, are only recently being understood or acknowledged. Parental separation is virtually inevitable once a suspect living in a home where children are present, and that may last as long as the investigation: 18 to 24 months in many cases if the couple are reconciled, or be permanent if they are not. Of course, the moral responsibility for all of the harms caused rests with the viewer of CSAM, but it is not uncommon for state agencies to resolve, or seek to ameliorate the problems that are caused to children by their parents, and there ought not be an exception to that principle here. These difficulties are known and foreseeable, and agencies which intervene in families to manage one set of harms need to take responsibility for managing any problems they unintentionally cause. Like Semmelweiss's surgeons, once the causes of inadvertent harms have been identified, practice has to change.

Potential solutions

In considering solutions, I hope the reader will indulge a brief description of what might be termed the 'Goldilocks principles' that might apply here, which is to say that a balance needs be struck between a vague or tokenistic view of safeguarding which over emphasises direct sexual risk and is purblind to secondary harms, and a naïve approach which focuses solely on the risk of suicide and incorporates a short term consideration including resolving the criminal matter and thereafter leaving the family to fend for themselves. A 'just right' approach considers and investigates the potential direct sexual risk posed by the father and offers support to the family whether that risk is potent or not. This would involve an early and comprehensive forensic examination of the suspect's devices, and a clinical assessment of his conduct. A family safety plan, negotiated with the family, may allow contact to take place between the father and children, and ultimately allow for family reconstitution if that is safe and desired. Services to help the mother and children navigate the extraordinarily stressful months following 'the knock' need to be provided.

There are police forces that have effectively institutionalised a consideration of secondary harms into their operations. Lincolnshire Constabulary employs a police officer who acts as a family liaison, and has no investigative role at all; his sole purpose is to keep the family informed and counselled. Other forces such as Thames Valley and West Mercia engage families using an independent support service. The Lucy Faithfull Foundation has been operating a helpline through its Stop it Now! arm since 2002, and therapeutic groups for viewers of CSAM and their partners have been delivered by that organisation operation for nearly two decades. Suicide reduction is one of the primary and realised goals of Stop it Now!. Talking Forward has operated a peer support group for women since 2022, and a number of self-directed and self-supporting groups are emerging who provide the sort of camaraderie that other organisations cannot. 'Writing Strong' is operated by way of the site anniehopewriter.wixsite.com, which supports women by engaging them in creative writing, and another, 'The world according to the knock', which can be found on X, provides advice and support.

Conclusion

The essential conclusions here are that the secondary harms brought into being by necessary police action can be ameliorated; they are unintended but foreseeable. It is unconscionable to accept them as immutable, and to simply blame them upon the suspect, which leaves children and women in a state of trauma with no relief. Systems dealing with these issues need to be informed about them and develop policies to deal with them. Individual therapists or counsellors dealing with women in these situations need to be aware of the substantial pressures exerted upon them by their partner, the agencies involved in their lives, the wider society and by their having to take responsibility for the outcomes of choices made by a trusted other.

References

APA (2018) American Dictionary of Psychology. https://dictionary.apa.org/.

Armitage R., Wager, N., Hudspith, L., Wibberley, D., & Gall, V. (2022). *We're not allowed to have experienced trauma. We're not allowed to go through the grieving process – Exploring the indirect harms associated with Child Sexual Abuse Material (CSAM) offending and its impacts on non-offending family members. Victims and Offenders.* Routledge: Open Access. doi.org/10.1080/15564886.2023.2172504.

Armitage, R., Wager, N., Wibberley, D., Hudspith, L., Efthymiadou E. & Gall, V. (2023) *The indirect harm of online child sexual abuse: the impact on families of people who offend.* The Faithfull Papers. https://www.lucyfaithfull.org.uk/faithfull-papers-research.htm.

Centre of Expertise on Child Sexual Abuse (2023) *Managing risk and trauma after online sexual offending.* csacentre.org.uk/research-resources/practice-resources/managing-risk-and-trauma-after-online-sexual-offending/.

Centre for Disease Control (1998) www.cdc.gov/violenceprevention/aces/about.

Families Outside (2016) *Picking up the Pieces. Support for Families of People Convicted of a Sexual Offence.* Barnados, Stop it Now! https://www.familiesoutside.org.uk/picking-pieces-2/.

Finkelhor, D. (1986) *A Sourcebook on Child Sexual Abuse.* Sage Publications.

Grant, H. (2023, 4 December) Thousands of UK young people caught watching online child abuse images. *The Guardian.*

Harris, D, Sheath, M, & Shields, R. (2024) First, do no harm: Critically revisiting contemporary approaches to child sexual abuse prevention. *Child Abuse & Neglect,* 153 (July).

James, B. (2009) *Treating Traumatized Children: New Insights and Creative Interventions.* Free Press.

Janoff-Bulman R. (1992) *Shattered Assumptions.* Free Press.

Martins, C., Godycki-Cwirko, M., Heleno, B, & J. (2018) Quaternary prevention: reviewing the concept. *European Journal of General Practice.* doi:10.1080/13814788.2017.1422177.

Parkes, C. M. (2009) *Love and Loss. The Roots of Grief and its Complications.* Routledge.

Semmelweiss, I. (1858) *The Etiology of Childbed Fever.* Orvosi Hetilap.

Sentencing Council for England and Wales (2002) https://www.gov.uk/government/organisations/the-sentencing-council-for-england-and-wales/about.

Sheath, M. (2022) *Crossing the Line.* Aspect Press.

Smallbone, S., Marshall, W. L., & Wortley, R. (2013) *Preventing Child Sexual Abuse, Evidence, Policy and Practice.* Taylor & Francis.

Stubley, A. (2015) 'He's a family man, but this is a dark side of him that I didn't know about': The lived experience of internet offenders' partners. Unpublished doctoral dissertation. Teeside University.

Weiss, D. S. & Marmar, C. R. (1997). The Impact of Event Scale-Revised. In J. P. Wilson & T. M. Keane (eds) *Assessing Psychological Trauma and PTSD: A Practitioner's Handbook* (pp. 399–411). Guilford Press.

Chapter 4

Social work assessment and response to primary and secondary child victims

An examination of risk assessment, safety planning and relationships within a context of shock, stress and trauma

Emma Barwell and Louise Wilcox

Introduction

What happens when an allegation of child abuse, or a report of concern, is made to the local authority's social services? How do social services and other agencies make decisions that potentially have a significant, even a life-changing, impact upon the circumstances of a child and their family? Are social services too harsh? Do they over-react? Is it fair to remove children from their parents, from the only home they have ever known? And why should we refer men who view child abuse material (CSAM) online? These are valid and understandable questions, asked not only by members of the public, but also by other professionals, even social workers.

Sometimes, it can feel as though the processes used to address child protection are shrouded in mystery and secrecy. Personal details and family courts are necessarily confidential. However, the statutory framework used by the local authority is publicly available and all professionals working with children and families should have a basic working knowledge of that legislation and related guidance. In this chapter the authors, who have a combined 50 years of social work experience, explain how social workers and their safeguarding partners respond when a referral is made to social services.

We need to be clear, before discussing social work intervention further, that social workers do not have the power, in and of themselves, to remove children from parents' care. Only the court via an order, or a police inspector using police protection (discussed below), can authorise the removal of children from the care of their parent or legal guardian, the person who has parental responsibility (PR) in law. Local authorities are the government at a local level, therefore, by default, registered social workers employed by local authorities function as agents of the State. It is in this capacity that social workers execute court orders giving authority to remove children, not by virtue of being a qualified social worker.

DOI: 10.4324/9781003509103-5

Statutory guidance

Social work in the UK is framed by civil law and grounded in the Children Act 1989. This Act is supported and enhanced by the Children Act 2004 and the Children and Social Work Act 2017. All three Acts of Parliament are interpreted by statutory guidance: working together to safeguard children. The guidance details how relevant agencies must work together to respond to child protection concerns by interpreting and applying the core requirements of statute. Therapists and other professionals can view their local authority's safeguarding procedures online via a simple search for their geographical region, or where the child is residing.

The Children Act 1989 enshrined key principles in relation to child protection and statutory intervention. The most well-known is the commitment to the paramountcy of the child's welfare, obliging the Court to consider the child's welfare above every other factor, in both public and private law. The 2004 Act expanded upon those principles by requiring all agencies, not just the Court and social services, to consider child protection in their functions, and the Social Work Act 2017 amended some of the 1989 Act, for example by creating Child Death Reviews and a regulatory body just for social workers. Notwithstanding the changes of the two subsequent Acts, the principles of the 1989 Act stand. These principles frame and guide the work of social services, in their assessment, safety planning and decision making, as a sole agency and in partnership with safeguarding partners.

Frequently, civil law is enacted alongside criminal law. For example, the police may investigate whether an allegation of child abuse meets the threshold for a criminal investigation, a situation about which the Crown Prosecution Service (CPS) will decide about charges, based on the standard of evidence and whether there is a realistic prospect of a conviction (as discussed in Chapter 5). At the same time, the local authority children's social care department may be gathering information about the same case but will be working on the balance of probability relating to potential risk of harm to that child. Although the outcome of the police investigation may result in a 'no further action' (NFA) decision, based on the available evidence, children's social care may still make applications to court to safeguard the child as the threshold for the risk of significant harm may have been met. Therapists must remain mindful that an NFA outcome from police does not automatically rule out risk of harm towards a child.

Historically, most referrals made to children's social care were allegations about a particular child being abused. However, local authorities are seeing an increasing number of referrals regarding online abuse, a significant rise, during and post-Covid.

In 2022 the National Centre for Missing & Exploited Children (NCMEC) received over 32 million reports from the public, containing nearly 88.3 million images and videos.

(Home Office, 2024)

The increased referrals include adults – most typically men within a family – viewing child sexual abuse material online (CSAM) and/or having sexual communication with a child. In more recent years, peer-on-peer/child-on-child abuse and 'self-generated' images (where children have been coerced, threatened or groomed to take images or perform via livestream) have been appearing, leading to a sharp rise in material being available.

Many families question why a referral to Children's Social Care is made when an offence online takes place. One research study identified a need for both primary and secondary victims of online viewing to be considered during an investigation, as they found that 57% of 127 CSAM offenders admitted to contact child abuse offending (disclosing 272 victims, of whom only 97 were identified and offered support (Bourke et. al., 2015)). Other considerations include the child in the home inadvertently seeing inappropriate or abusive material. Even if a child victim cannot be positively identified at the point of arrest, such a situation would constitute an appropriate expression of concern. Therefore, the matter must be investigated, online victims identified and approached and the safety and welfare of possible secondary victims assured.

Throughout this chapter, composite case studies will be used to illustrate client stories. These may resonate with the work you are carrying out.

The initial response to a report of concern or a referral to social services

Many children's social care departments now take a multi-disciplinary approach to assessing referrals at the first point of contact. These front door services are usually known as Multi-Agency Safeguarding Hubs, or MASH teams. MASH teams review each referral from a health, police and children's social care perspective, screening for risk of harm to a child and deciding about a response, whether that be no further action, signposting to another service or being sent to a social worker for assessment. Sometimes, the decision might be that there is no need for statutory intervention at the point of referral, perhaps because the threshold for intervention has not been met, or sometimes because the family have already taken protective action. If it is felt there is an immediate risk of significant harm to a child, a multi-agency (strategy) meeting will be convened to decide about next steps.

Case study 1

A father who has parental responsibility (PR), but who is not living with his children, has contact with them every weekend. He has been arrested for viewing online child abuse material (CSAM). The mother ceased contact as soon as she became aware of the arrest. This is being challenged formally by father, who seeks a Child Arrangement Order (Contact Order) from the family court. The police referred the matter to social services. Social services consider that the mother has taken appropriate action in immediately ceasing contact and therefore there is currently no direct risk to the children. Social services may await the court's decision before deciding whether there is a role for them.

Strategy discussion

The first action of the response to a referral is to judge whether there is a risk of harm, e.g. that a child has suffered or may suffer significant harm. Social services are responsible for convening the meeting, which must be held within one working day (or on the same day as receipt of referral if imminent risk is suspected) and must be chaired by a children's social care manager. Representatives from both the police and relevant health services should also attend, as well as other agencies as relevant; for example, if the child attends a nursery, representatives should attend the meeting, as should the health visitor. The purpose of the meeting is to share available information, to discuss and agree whether the referral has met the threshold for a child protection investigation and if it has, whether that investigation will be by only social services (single agency investigation), or as a joint investigation with the police. Although it is always best practice for families to be informed that a referral has been received and a strategy meeting convened, should it be viewed as placing a child at increased risk of harm, the meeting can go ahead without parents being informed and/or without gaining their consent.

The core attendees at the meeting must agree next steps, and whether it is felt the information shared reaches the threshold for a child protection investigation, commonly referred to as a Section 47 [of the Children Act 1989]. This allows the local authority and police to carry out further inquiries and then make a decision as to whether the investigation will be children's social care led, police led or a joint investigation. As discussed above, either the police or children's social care may continue involvement when the other closes a case. All children in the household and those outside, where risk of harm may be relevant, will be considered at the meeting. For example, should a man be arrested for viewing child abuse images online and he is known to have contact with nieces and nephews under the age of 18, they will be included in decision making. If the adult of interest works with children, for example teachers, social workers, care workers, or medics, the local authority designated officer, commonly referred to as the LADO, would also be involved. In such cases, the LADO will provide advice to the employer and sometimes oversee a case.

In the event of the strategy discussion agreeing that the referral does not meet the threshold for investigation, social services may carry out an assessment to gain more information to help to decide about further intervention or support, for example for implementing a child in need plan (CIN plan – see below) as opposed to a child protection plan, or immediate steps to remove and safeguard. If the strategy meeting has decided that a child is at risk of significant harm, or may have been harmed, what happens next?

Direct emergency risk to a child

Should the strategy meeting identify an immediate risk to the child's life or limb, there are two options for intervention: police protection (PP) or an Emergency Protection Order (EPO). Police protection is a power available only to the police and allows them to immediately remove a child from a parent's care, on an emergency basis, for a period of up to 72 hours. The PP must be authorised at inspector level, although it may be implemented by officers on the ground at the location of the relevant child. The PP does not need to last for 72 hours but cannot last for longer than 72 hours.

An Emergency Protection Order is exactly as described and allows for the immediate, summary removal of a child from their parents' care. Gaining an EPO relies on Court availability, so PP may be used as an interim measure to keep a child safe, if a Court hearing cannot be held, for example, until the day after the serious risk has been identified. Removing a child from their home without warning or planning is a serious, some might say draconian measure, and to be used only when there is an immediate threat to a child's life, or a risk of serious injury. An EPO lasts for eight days but may be extended up to 15 days to allow the local authority to further plan for the child's welfare if necessary. Out-of-hours EPOs are heard by duty magistrates.

Risk of significant harm identified

In the event of a risk of significant harm being identified without an immediate threat to a child's life or welfare, the strategy meeting will arrange a child protection investigation (S47 enquiry).

> A Section 47 enquiry refers to Section 47 of the Children Act 1989 and involves social workers gathering evidence and speaking with the child, family and other relevant professionals to determine if any interventions may be beneficial to the child's welfare.
>
> (NSPCC, 2024)

Social services must work in partnership with parents, unless doing so may increase or create a risk to a child (another of the key principles from the 1989 Act).

Section 47 also refers to the legal capacity for dispensing with parental consent, if necessary, in the course of carrying out a child protection investigation, so allows the local authority, or the police, to contact agencies to enquire about a child's welfare as part of their investigation: for example, social services may request information about a child's health from their GP, or health visitor, or speak to the school. The time from an investigation starting (strategy meeting) to an initial child protection conference is 15 working days, should it be deemed a child has reached this threshold of risk of significant harm.

Case study 2

A 15-year-old girl tells her form teacher that she saw 'loads of weird photos' on her stepdad's desktop computer at home; that the photos are of her neighbour's three-year-old child naked in the paddling pool in the next-door garden. Some of the photos are of the little girl bending over, playing with a toy in the water. The teenage girl says her stepdad is 'creepy' and she never liked him. The school are aware that the teenager has a younger sister and call social services. Social services check their system to see that the stepfather has a conviction for viewing online child abuse images. A strategy discussion takes place regarding the teenage girl, her younger sister and the three-year-old child living next door. Because the photos are indecent and because the stepdad has a previous conviction, a S47 investigation (joint agency, i.e. social services and police) is agreed and other agencies are consulted to see if they have ever had concern about all three children.

Child protection conference and plan

A child protection conference comprises relevant agencies and is chaired by a local authority independent reviewing officer. The aim of the conference is to share relevant information and formulate a child protection plan (CP plan) for reducing the identified risk to a particular child or children. The conference should invite the parents/legal guardian to the conference, with the aim of working in partnership with them to help them to care more safely for their children and reduce the identified risk. Older children should also be invited to the conference and their views and wishes actively sought, if appropriate. The plan must be initially reviewed after three months and then six-monthly thereafter, working towards the CP plan being discharged and the case 'stepped down' to less intrusive support from the local authority.

Case study 3

A couple have two daughters, aged seven and nine. One day, the seven-year-old mentions to her teacher that daddy has a laptop under his desk and told her off when she tried to look at it. Two weeks later, the police contact the school to ask if there is any concern for the girls' welfare. The school say the children attended the nursery linked to the school, so have been known for several years and there has never been concern about them. The school also report that the parents engage normally. The police tell the school that child abuse images have been traced to father's laptop and he has been arrested. The images are of teenage girls, 13 years and older. A strategy discussion is held the same day and the school attend. At the discussion, it is agreed that father will be asked to vacate the family home for the duration of the police investigation and whilst an assessment is conducted to assess any risk to his daughters. Initially, the mother struggles to accept this, but the father does agree to move to his relative's house (the police and social services confirm that the relative has no under-18 children living in his home and none who visit). There is no indication that the girls have been harmed, however, there is agreement that they may be at risk of harm. Therefore, an initial child protection conference is booked and a safety plan put in place that until the conference, there will be no contact between father and daughters, subject to planned and un-announced social work visits, until the outcome of assessments. The father is bailed and at the conference contact arrangements are put in place whilst assessments are undertaken.

Ongoing work and safety planning

A safety plan is designed to address immediate and perhaps medium-term risk (it might be revised in the future to address a longer-term risk as necessary) and lays out how professionals and family members will work together to keep children safe, stipulating who will carry out which actions. Frequently, the safety plan will be a voluntary arrangement, entered into by all parties. There is no standard template for this and each Local Authority will work within their own practice framework. Good practice requires safety planning at the start of the investigation/ assessment process and will be strength-based, clear and achievable. Therefore, in our example above, we prepare and mitigate risk at the beginning of the casework relationship, until we know otherwise via assessment. We do not wait until the outcome of the assessment to learn whether the girls are at risk of harm, and then put in safety measures.

A good safety plan acknowledges that risk is dynamic and that urgent change may be needed in response to an increase in risk or new investigation information being shared. However, generally, any amendments to the plan should be made at the review child protection conference. The plan should also be shared with all relevant parties, even if not directly participating in the plan.

No risk of significant harm identified

In the event of the child protection investigation concluding there is no risk of significant harm to the child, the case may be closed, referred to 'early-help' services, or the family may be offered a child in need plan (CIN plan).

Child in need

Under Section 17 of the Children Act 1989, a child will be considered in need if:

- They are unlikely to achieve or maintain or to have the opportunity to achieve or maintain a reasonable standard of health or development without provision of services from the Local Authority.
- Their health or development is likely to be significantly impaired, or further impaired, without the provision of services from the Local Authority.
- They have a disability.

Some examples of children in need might be an asylum-seeking child, or a child who has Special Educational Needs and Disabilities.

The local authority has a duty to meet the needs of every child in their area, even if the child is not normally resident within a local authority. The local authority in which the child is located at the point of the need being identified must meet the need, if only initially.

In the same way that a child protection conference will create a plan, a child in need plan will be put together, but always with the consent of the parent and child (if appropriate). Agencies involved will be invited to child in need meetings, where the plan will be reviewed and support offered. This is a voluntary process for families but it is always best that families and professional agencies work together, when concern for a child's wellbeing has been identified.

Case study 4

A single mother is the sole carer for her nine-year-old disabled son. She meets his personal care needs, including changing incontinence pads and bathing. The child attends a special needs school. The school have told the mother they believe it inappropriate for her to continue to provide her son's personal care and the mother is worried about being accused of sexual abuse. The school refer the matter to the local authority. After assessment, the local authority concludes there is no risk to the son from mother and put together a child in need plan (CIN plan). This helps mother to ensure she is receiving all relevant income and support, including support with personal care.

Why are we worried about men who view online child sexual abuse images?

It is our view that the matter of an adult viewing online child sexual abuse images (CSAM) should be an automatic referral to social services and the police. If a therapist is made aware of ongoing viewing of CSAM, undetected by the police, then this should be taken to supervisors for specialist support, as well as seeking advice and guidance from their professional and/or governing body with the possibility of disclosure in mind (please see Chapter 16 for a legal analysis around therapeutic disclosure). This may feel counter-intuitive for counsellors and psychotherapists, whose relationship with their client is one of trust. In our opinion, there are robust reasons for the need to refer:

1. It is illegal. The Protection of Children Act 1978 made it an offence for anyone to make, distribute, show, or advertise indecent images of children under 18 years of age. This does not correlate with the age of sexual consent in the UK, which is 16 years, so it is imperative for professionals working with children to understand the requirements of the 1978 Act and the difference in the age of consent. The Protection of Children Act stipulates that 18 is the age below which a child cannot consent to sexual or indecent images being made of them and subsequently distributed. A court in 2003 found that causing an image to be displayed on a screen amounted to making it (CPS, 2020), so live-streaming, whether pay-by-view, in chat rooms or even using images that children have made of themselves, also amounts to making and distributing indecent images of children.

2. The male watching or viewing child sexual abuse material (CSAM) online may have access to children in their offline world. Generally, early research about males who view child abuse images online indicates that the risk of contact abuse is low, as is the risk of re-offending. However, low risk does not mean no risk. Due to the endemic rise in the global distribution of child sexual abuse material, researchers across continents have joined forces to work together to understand the true scale and nature of this crime and to challenge some findings in earlier literature. The Finish Organisation Suojellaan Lapsia, Protect Children, carried out anonymous surveys via the dark web, for those actively

seeking child sexual abuse online. The ReDirection Survey Report (2021) found CSAM is increasingly live streamed and that many users of the material have also abused, or thought about abusing, in their offline world, resulting in hybrid offenders and victims.

> 52% of respondents have felt afraid that viewing CSAM might lead to sexual acts against a child. . . . 44% of respondents said that viewing CSAM made them think about seeking direct contact with children. . . . 37% of respondents have sought direct contact with children after viewing CSAM.
>
> (ReDirection Survey Report, 2021, p.16)

Risk relating to sexual harm considers many factors which, when combined, can create an offending template as unique as the individual the social worker is assessing. Criteria linked to offending pathways can include previous anti-social or criminal behaviour, child abuse or neglect on the part of the client, previous contact abuse, and ease of access to children (London Safeguarding Children Partnership, 2022). Counsellors and psychotherapists interact with their client in the room and must necessarily rely on self-referred clients to provide all relevant information.

Referrals from external agencies. Often, referrals from external agencies (for example from a GP or charity) about the presenting matter may not contain all information pertinent to the client's offending history. It is likely that unless a referral for counselling is made by a statutory body for a specific purpose, which necessitates the disclosure of relevant facts, therapists will be reliant on their client to share information relating to their online behaviour.

Access to external information. Social workers, on the other hand, in the context of a child protection investigation or assessment, can access information about previous criminality and family structure, as well as social interactions, allowing for a full risk assessment that considers all relevant factors. Therefore, police and social services will know, or be able to uncover, whether the client has access to children in the client's offline world and can risk assess and safety plan accordingly, using safeguarding partners to help to monitor and mitigate the risk of harm to children.

Manipulation. Adults who abuse or harm children often demonstrate the ability to manipulate others and this is present in their offending patterns, for example, overcoming external barriers by lying to partners about their online content, viewing images once partners have gone to bed, setting up passwords to protect their saved images or downloading software to access information on the dark web. These patterns are incontrovertible and demonstrated time and again by case reviews and case histories. Online and offline abusers manipulate the children involved. Historically, the image of 'grooming' a child was painted as taking place over an extensive period and various models were created to show the strategies used to captivate and sustain the abuse, adapting findings from research such as De Santisteban et al. (2018). However, recent research has shown how the internet has intensified and evolved the ability to harm children at speed. The WeProtect Global Alliance's 2023 Global Threat Assessment found that the average time for a child to be 'locked into' a grooming conversation was 45 minutes: the shortest time found was 19 seconds, with just seven questions.

Be vigilant. The need for continued professional curiosity and vigilance cannot be over-stated for all professionals who work with males who view child sexual abuse imagery. Some men who view such images may absolutely desire help and will commit to the therapy process, but we cannot assume that they will disclose further, relevant information to a professional. And we, as professionals, cannot assume that we will recognise lies, obfuscation or denial on the part of our client. The very nature of abuse is to deceive. All of us, professional or no, are vulnerable to these dynamics, and to being groomed.

3. For the photos or live streaming to take place real children have been, or are being, abused. For child sexual abuse material to be available, children have been abused, or are being abused in real time, during live streaming and in chat rooms. This is not a victimless crime. Children repeatedly report the long-lasting impact, evident in the Our Voice (2024) survey for survivors of sexual violence in childhood.

> In a Canadian Centre for Child Protection survey, nearly 70% of CSAM survivors said that the distribution of their images impacts them differently than the hands-on abuse they suffered as the distribution never ends and the images are permanent.
>
> (ReDirection Survey Report, 2021)

Due to the increased availability of technology and its use across our lives, children as young as three years old have been creating 'self-generated' imagery that has been captured and distributed as child sexual abuse material. In 2023, the UK based Internet Watch Foundation analysed material they intercepted for the first time, showing children between the ages of three and six years who fell into this category. They note the term 'self-generated' can be interpreted as victim-blaming language, which can increase the minimisation of harm by those who have offended, as well as their partners and others, stating, 'children are not responsible for their own sexual abuse'. In the 2,401 self-generated images in this age range, 91% were girls; 15% showed penetration of themselves, or others.

Sextortion is another growing area of concern, following the online sexual abuse that has taken place. An experiential video of this, by the National Centre for Missing and Exploited Children, can be viewed online (The No Escape Room), and can help to fully understand the pressure and consequences for adolescents in today's world.

Assessing risk. Children's safety is a priority for the police and social services. Therapists hearing client disclosure about viewing child sexual abuse material should take advice about reporting from their professional body, or from the StopSO Board members (see Chapter 16). Continuous risk assessment, as well as appropriate challenge, should form part of the therapist's agenda when working with males who view child abuse material. In the wider context of preventing online viewing, the relationship of trust between therapist and client is crucially important in bringing about necessary change, and in some cases, with support, it may be possible to bring the client to a point of self-reporting. However, ultimately, the welfare of children is a matter for all professionals involved in any aspect of child protection. With this in mind, regulating bodies and professional supervision are the first port of call for therapists who have to manage the issues or concerns that may arise.

Case study 5

Jeremy is in his mid-50s and has hired a female psychotherapist because he needed help with long-standing sex addiction. He said the problem started when he was about 17 years old and he has always had an active sex life, often having multiple partners at once. After the menopause, his wife 'lost interest in sex'. He increasingly used the internet for pornography and paid younger woman for sex, often women in their early 20s. As the therapeutic relationship progressed, Jeremy mentioned that he found 'teenage women' on the internet more stimulating and had joined chat rooms to watch live-streamed sex. The therapist uncovered that some of the girls involved in the live streaming were under-18 years old. Jeremy assured the therapist the girls 'look like they're enjoying it' and are 'definitely' not being coerced. Five months into his therapy, Jeremy did not arrive for his appointment. Several days later, his therapist reads in the local newspaper that he had been arrested for watching live streaming of young girls being abused.

Conclusion

This chapter has examined the different possible responses by social care to child protection referrals, with a particular focus on referrals about children who are the victims of adult males viewing online child abuse. We have also discussed the reasons for the high level of concern about the crime of viewing online child sexual abuse material (CSAM). As we note, viewing CSAM is not a victimless crime and therapists' professional bodies will advise members about referral to statutory services. Taking such action may feel counter-intuitive, a betrayal even, of the therapeutic relationship and the trust of the client; a difficult place with potential for conflict, not only in the relationship with the client, but perhaps internally for the therapist, too.

Notwithstanding that conflict, referring to statutory services is, in our opinion, the only way to try to ensure the identification and future protection of the children in the images, and it is the only way to assess risk to any children in the male's offline world, because all the children involved must be identified and safeguarded, whether they be the primary or secondary victims. Adult men who view child abuse images need help and support to prevent further offending, but the immediate safety of the children involved should be the priority for all professionals.

References

Bourke, M. L., Fragomeli, L., Detar, P. J., Sullivan, M. A., Meyle, E., & O'Riordan, M. (2015) The use of tactical polygraph with sex offenders. *Journal of Sexual Aggression,* 21(3), 354–367.

Children Act (1989) https://www.legislation.gov.uk/ukpga/1989/41/contents.

Children Act (2004) https://www.legislation.gov.uk/ukpga/2004/31/contents.

Children and Social Work Act (2014) https://www.legislation.gov.uk/ukpga/2014/6/contents.

Children and Social Work Act (2017) https://www.legislation.gov.uk/ukpga/2017/16/contents.

Crown Prosecution Service (2020) Indecent and Prohibited Images of Children. https://www.cps.gov.uk/legal-guidance/indecent-and-prohibited-images-children.

De Santisteban, P., Del Hoyo, J., Alcázar-Córcoles, M. Á. & Gámez-Guadix, M. (2018) Progression, maintenance, and feedback of online child sexual grooming: A qualitative analysis of online predators. *Child Abuse and Neglect*, 80, 203–215. doi:10.1016/j.chiabu.2018.03.026.

Home Office (2024) Child Abuse Image Database (CAID) Empowering Law Enforcement through technology to protect children and identify offenders of child sexual abuse and exploitation. https://assets.publishing.service.gov.uk/media/6644af2d993111924d9d3550/CAID_Brochure_May2024.pdf.

London Safeguarding Children Partnership (2022) *London Safeguarding Children Procedures*, 7th ed., CP10. Risk Management of Known Offenders. https://www.londonsafeguardingchildrenprocedures.co.uk/risk_manag_offend.html.

National Centre for Missing and Exploited Children (n.d.) No Escape Room: Launches with new data: Interactive Experience Exposes Dangers of Financial Sextortion. https://www.missingkids.org/blog/2024/no-escape-room-launches-with-interactive-experience.

NSPCC (2024) Child Protection System in England. https://learning.nspcc.org.uk/child-protection-system/england#:~:text=A%20Section%2047%20enquiry%20refers,beneficial%20to%20the%20child's%20welfare.

Our Voice (2024) Survey for survivors of sexual violence in childhood. https://www.ourvoicesurvey.com/survey/english.

ReDirection Survey Report (2021) Suojellaan Lapsia: Protect Children. CSAM Users in the Dark Web: Protecting Children Through Prevention. https://www.suojellaanlapsia.fi/en/redirection

WeProtect: Global Alliance. Global Threat Assessment (2023) Assessing the Scale and Scope of Child Sexual Abuse Online. https://www.weprotect.org/global-threat-assessment-23/.

Working together to safeguard children (2024) Department of Education. https://www.gov.uk/government/publications/working-together-to-safeguard-children—2.

Chapter 5

The pathway through the criminal justice system before and after conviction

Glyn Hudson-Allez

Introduction

When clients first attend for therapy after getting the knock, despite having a solicitor to guide them through the process, they are full of uncertainty with questions regarding what they might anticipate will happen to them. Therapists having some understanding of the general criminal justice procedures can help allay these some of these fears to allow the therapeutic process to commence. This chapter will cover the roles of the police, probation, duty solicitors, social workers if children are involved (following on from the previous chapter), courses available to the client from other organisations like the Lucy Faithfull Foundation, MAPPA meetings and post-conviction supervisory roles of the police liaison officers following the community integration plans. Some of this chapter will inter-relate to Chapter 4.

The criminal justice system

The criminal justice system is an adversarial system, so not specifically a search for truth (Hudson-Allez, 2004), but a battle between two sides (two adversaries). It has suffered over the years by a lack of central government overview of long-term strategies, underfunding, with legal policies often developed in response to high-profile criminal events to appease the media and grieving/outraged victims and their families (Hudson-Allez, 2014; Zilney, 2021), without considering the collateral damage impacting the wider familial network of an offender (Hudson-Allez, 2023). See also Chapter 3 overviewing the unintended consequences of the knock, leading to the secondary victimisation of families and their children. It is not proposed here to provide an overview of the ministerial responsibilities within the criminal justice system, but to provide the therapist with an overview of the process that the client who has committed a sexual offence may become locked into.

The police investigation

How does it all start? There are 39 police forces assigned specific territories throughout England, four in Wales, one in Scotland (Police Scotland) and one in

DOI: 10.4324/9781003509103-6

Northern Ireland (PSNI). These forces have a certain amount of independence in how they conduct their policing activities, although they cannot be independent of the law. Therefore, when referring to police activities, we will state the general case, although it is necessary to be mindful that not all forces act in a uniform manner. Police forces have special investigative teams to deal with online sexual offenders, often called POLIT (Police Online Investigation Team), but many forces will also have specialist teams for investigating child abuse, adult and elder sexual assault, historical sexual abuse, organised criminal sexual activities and MOSOVO Teams (the Management of Sexual Offenders and Violent Offenders). The reader here will notice the anomaly that many of our online offender clients, who are viewers of child sexual abuse material (CSAM) yet may never leave the comfort of their own homes, are linked together with violent offenders.

The investigation usually begins from intelligence received, either from the public who are worried about the activities of an individual, a partner who discovers inappropriate material on her husband's phone or computer, a child who discloses inappropriate behaviour at home or school or from the technical investigations of other people that may be discovered when examining the IP addresses from other devices. This is a burgeoning criminal issue, and for the period 2020–21, the numbers of victims reporting online abuse had increased by 400% (Skidmore & Aitkenhead, 2022), whereas the NSPCC argue it is 79% over the five years between 2017–2022 (NSPCC, 2024).

The investigative teams also have many undercover police officers searching the internet, particularly in chat rooms pretending to be children to lure or 'out' potential offenders. They will encourage conversation with their target, and once they feel the conversation is meaningful, *i.e.* sexual, they will drop into the conversation that they are underage. If the conversation continues, then the person will get 'the knock', a police investigation into their activities and devices. Under English law, entrapment is not a defence, although it is considered to be an abuse of its process and may lead to a trial failing. In these circumstances, the police will rely on finding evidence of the person viewing CSAM on their devices for a prosecution to succeed.

There are also vigilante groups online, self-appointed paedophile hunters, who create fake social media accounts, again posing as underage children. The number of police cases brought as a result of these paedophile-hunting organisations had tripled in two years (BBC News, 2019). These sting operations may involve hours/days/months of targeting an individual into inappropriate conversations or arranging to meet 'a child', so they have a lot invested in 'bringing the person to justice' under their right to a citizen's arrest, to advertise it widely on social media by recording and publishing the arrest, which inflicts personal harm on the individual and his family (in secondary victimisation discussed in Chapter 3), long before he has been found guilty under the law. These confrontations sometimes result in false imprisonment when an alleged offender has tried to escape, and even physical violence between them, and again, the argument of entrapment needs to be considered. However, there is no law against these vigilante groups conducting their activities, so it can be argued that the State colludes with them.

The knock

If police feel there is sufficient evidence to initiate an investigation, the individual will receive the knock, a home visit from the police. After obtaining warrants from the magistrate's court, in some forces, this will be a discrete visit with two detectives not uniform. In other cases, this will be a six-person uniformed early morning raid, sometimes with dogs, with blue lights flashing outside to notify the neighbourhood, promoting distress for all the occupants inside. Some forces will triage at the home premises the computer devices and/or phones deemed to be considered through which the offences have taken place. Others may seize any and all devices considered pertinent to their investigation, which may mean devices belonging to the partner, lodger or the children of the alleged offender, or anyone else who lives within the house. The alleged offender will be removed from the property and taken to the police station for an initial interview.

At the police station, if the individual does not have a lawyer, a duty solicitor can be requested for the interview, who may attend in person or online through the interview. They most commonly will advise the person to respond 'no comment' to the questioning, until they both have an understanding of the potential charges, to prevent the alleged offender from incriminating themselves. After the interview, they often are kept overnight in a cell and released in the morning with bail conditions. These conditions will usually require a monthly, or three-monthly, revisit to the police station. If further enquiries need to be made, the individual can be re-bailed for a further three months. The maximum length of time a person can be on bail is 12 months without being charged, but this generally requires approval from a magistrate. However, there is such a backlog with so many of these cases now, that they are often 'released under investigation', which means they do not have to repeatedly attend the police station, but the same restrictions apply. If the allegations involve the person viewing child sexual abuse material (CSAM) online, a condition will be that they are not to be alone in the presence of a child under the age of 18. So, although a man is supposed to be considered innocent until proven guilty, this does not apply to alleged sexual offences. If the alleged offender has children of his own, the social services safeguarding team will be notified (see Chapter 4 for details of the procedure), who will also attend and advise the person that they cannot return home to their wife/partner or children. If they have no personal resources to rent somewhere, it often involves the person asking to stay with family or sofa-surf. Some may even take to the streets; such is the extent of their shame. One can see how mental health breakdown and potential suicidality is common in these alleged offenders.

Part of the investigative knock will also be to attend their place of employment to seize their work computer. This obviously informs the employer and all work colleagues of the alleged offences, and invariably they lose their employment, creating a further financial burden on themselves and family in having to support two homes, and without savings will require support of universal credit. The social services safeguarding team will visit the wife/partner, and demand that the children are told of the offences, and also will inform the children's school. Some forces are now developing a Victim Support Officer role to liaise, advise and support the family of an alleged offender, but these are in the minority of forces. Mostly, the arrested person and his family are left unsupported in a state they describe as limbo, as the criminal justice process slowly grinds its way along, which may mean years.

The forensic investigation

Most forces have a high-tech crime unit, or its equivalent, where the devices are digitally forensically examined. This involves using software that exactly mirrors all the hard drives of the devices, allowing thorough examination without the contamination of the evidence. The software has specific algorithms with multi-modal image or video descriptors (Lee et al., 2023) to speed up the process of detecting CSAM which may have hundreds and thousands of images on just one device. All imagery, whether still photographs or videos, will be examined and details recorded, with CSAM being categorised: A, penetrative (the most serious), B, sexual activity, C, erotica. Greater challenges are involved in examining live-streaming events, but again software has been developed to provide evidence of activity (Horseman, 2018). Even if the imagery were originally thumbnails and subsequently deleted by the person under investigation, these deleted images will still be included in the count that goes on the charge sheet. The Online Safety Act of 2023 has reclassified some of the charges, including cyberflashing, which is sending unsolicited pictures of one's genitals ('dick-pics') with the intent of causing distress.

When investigations are completed, which may take up to a year, depending on the complexity of the investigation, the investigative police usually call the alleged offender back to the police station for a second interview, to see if any further evidence can be gathered, and to inform the person of the proposed charges, before sending the details to the Crown Prosecution Service (CPS). The CPS will make the decision whether or not the alleged offender is to be charged on the basis of all the forensic evidence and witness statements gathered by the investigating police officers. The wait for this decision can vary between weeks and months. Sometimes the case is dropped at this stage if the CPS feel, on a cost-benefit analysis, there is an insufficient case to answer. This is called NFA: no further action. However, this might be a year or 18 months after first getting the knock, and the individuals will not regain all that they have lost: their marriage/partnership, their employment and lost income, their friendships and well-being within the community, and access to their children may still be denied.

Alternatively, if the CPS feel there is a case to answer, it is at this stage the person is formerly charged, through the post or possibly entailing another visit to the local police station. It is important to emphasise that being charged of an offence is not an establishment of guilt; they are still at this stage an alleged offender, and the onus is on the prosecution to demonstrate their guilt. There now is another lengthy delay waiting for a Court date.

The courts

The individuals' first appearance in court will be to a magistrate's court where they will indicate their plea of guilty or not guilty. If the person pleads 'guilty', the case will be adjourned for a pre-sentence report (PSR) from a probation officer, who, on the basis of a short interview, will determine an assessment of risk to the individual themselves and risk of re-offending. Magistrates can send offenders to prison for up to two years, but if the magistrate deems the case to be of sufficient seriousness to warrant a longer custodial sentence, as magistrates are not judges, the case will be adjourned (more delay) to Crown Court.

If the person pleads 'not guilty' at magistrate level, then again, the case will be adjourned to Crown Court for a trial with a jury. If found guilty, the trial will be adjourned for PSRs before sentencing. It is at this stage that a therapist who has been working with the defendant may be asked to write a letter or a report to help the judge determine the appropriate sentence to impose on the now convicted offender (see Chapter 17).

Probation pre-sentence reports (PSRs)

The probation service works with police and the courts to help manage people who have been convicted of an offence and assess their risk to themselves, the public, and their risk of reoffending. The service was privatised in 2015 under a scheme called Transforming Rehabilitation, which included a payment by results mechanism that was fundamentally flawed. It was returned to the public sector in 2021 after much chaos, but it meant a loss of good and experienced probation officers, and the skill set is still being built up, under conditions of a burgeoning caseload.

Pre-sentence reports are designed to provide a judge with expert assessment of the risk posed by an offender of reoffending, rehabilitative work undertaken and to make sentence recommendations. Probation officers may use a variety of different actuarial instruments to inform their assessment of risk of an offender: OASys (Offender Assessment System, but not specifically for sexual offenders); ARMS (McNaughton Nicholls & Webster, 2014) that identifies static, dynamic and protective risk factors specifically for sexual offenders; Risk Matrix 2000 (Thornton, 2002) that looks for indications of recidivism, and SARN (Structured Assessment of Risk and Need (Webster et al., 2006) that also looks for dynamic risk factors. However, using actuarial instruments alone is considered to be necessary (Grove et al., 2000) but insufficient for a thorough analysis of risk, and for sexual offenders, the gold standard would be The Sexual Violence Risk-20 (SVR-20) using a structured professional judgement process (Hart & Boer, 2021). However, the probation officers will argue that they have insufficient time to undertake this with a burgeoning case load, so they will opt for the quickest and easiest. Also there has been an increase in the number of PSRs delivered to court orally rather than in writing (which again takes less time for the probation officer) and a 22% increase of the number of sentences imposed without a PSR in place at all (Fouzder, 2018), which is significant if one considers that offenders are ten times more likely to get a community service order with a pre-sentence report.

Sentencing

As mentioned, magistrates most commonly impose the lighter sentences, but can send defendants to prison for up to two years. This may be required to be served immediately, or it may be suspended for a period of up to two years. This requires the defendant to maintain their good behaviour for the period of the suspension, or they will be sent to prison immediately. There are usually requirements of a suspended sentence: to attend probation weekly, rehabilitation activity requirements (RAR), community service, an electronic tag with a night-time curfew and perhaps a sex offender course like Horizon or Kaizen. The judge is most likely to suspend the sentence if there is a realistic prospect of rehabilitation in the community, with strong personal mitigation and a detrimental impact on others (*e.g.* dependents) if he goes to prison.

Magistrates may impose a community order that can be for six months to three years, and includes one-to-one supervision with a probation officer. A Sexual Harm Prevention Order (or Sexual Risk Order) will be imposed on all individuals convicted of a sexual offence, and the contents will depend on the recommendations of the probation officer after the evaluation of risk of harm to themselves and/or others and risk of reoffending. It may include powers for the police to make unannounced visits to check on the person's devices, and to restrict movements near vulnerable adults or children. They will also be placed on the sex offender's register automatically for between five and ten years (or life if sufficiently serious, although registrants can apply for a review of this) which requires the person to notify the Police Public Protection Unit (PPU) of their movements, particularly if being away from home for more than seven consecutive days. However, a meta-analysis reviewing 25 years of sexual offender registration and notification (SORN) evaluations has shown that SORN shows no statistical significance on recidivism of sexual and non-sexual offences (Zgoba & Mitchell, 2021).

A Notification Order (NO) requires individuals who have been convicted of a sexual offence overseas to notify the UK police on their return to the UK. They will then be placed on the SOR to become subject to notification requirements. The number of these orders has been increasing year on year suggesting more people who have been convicted overseas are returning to this country (Ministry of Justice, 2023).

Prison

If the person receives a prison sentence, they will be taken immediately from the court sentencing hearing to prison. In Scotland offenders are not sent to prison if their sentence is under 12 months. There are some prisons specifically for housing people convicted of sexual offences, like HMP Whatton, the largest in Europe. In other prisons, as people who commit sexual offences often have a difficult time due to being targeted and attacked by prison staff and other inmates, they are often separated into a dedicated wing called the Vulnerable Prisoner Unit (VPUs). With good behaviour, most will serve just half to two-thirds of their sentence in prison, and the rest served in the community 'under licence', although any minor infringement of the rules of their release set by probation will lead to their being recalled into prison for the remainder of their sentence.

In 2005, Imprisonment for Public Protection (IPP) was introduced into statute. This was originally designed to protect the public from dangerous criminals whose crimes did not merit a life sentence, and meant that irrespective of the length of jail sentence given by the court, the offenders were held in prison indefinitely. At the time, men who committed a sexual offence for the second time were automatically given an IPP. The IPP was abolished in 2012, but not reviewed retrospectively; 96% of these have not been released. One third have a tariff of four years or less but are still imprisoned, and complaints of overflowing prisons go unheard.

Horizon, iHorizon and Kaizen

Horizon is a treatment programme delivered to men who have committed a sexual offence and are deemed to be of medium, high or very high risk of reoffending, which could be conducted either in custodial or community settings. The focus was on men who either accepted responsibility for their offence, and those who maintained their innocence, or minimised the offence. This programme aims to provide a biopsychosocial model of change, building on the principles of the Risk Need and Responsivity (RNR) model (Andrews & Bonta, 2013), the Good Lives Model (GLM) (Ward, Mann & Gannon, 2007) and desistance from crime (Farmer, Beech & Ward, 2012). These courses are always conducted in groups and consist of 31 sessions over 62 hours. Some men respond well to them, enjoying the connection with other men who have been through similar experiences; others, particularly those on the autistic spectrum (who are a large proportion of StopSO forensic clients), struggle to work in groups, which may be interpreted by the facilitators as being resistant to rehabilitation. Ogloff et al. (2012) argued that it was short-sighted that these treatment programmes do not allow exploration of the participant's own childhood sexual victimisation or traumatic history considering they are five times more likely than the non-abused general population to commit an offence, with the strongest associations for sexual and violent offences.

iHorizon is an adaptation of the course specifically for individuals with online convictions, and not for contact offenders. This course is always conducted in the community and consists of 23 sessions over 46 hours. Both Horizon courses aim to cover the domains of:

- Managing life's problems
- Healthy thinking

- Healthy sexual interests
- Positive relationships
- Sense of purpose.

Elliott & Hambly (2023) undertook an assessment of both programmes and found a positive improvement in the participants, although they did not take account of extraneous factors (like personal therapy), nor did they conduct a randomly controlled trial, considered the gold-standard of outcome research.

Kaizen is a programme for offenders considered high or very high risk who have committed violent and/or contact sexual offences. Again, it is based on a strengths-based approach and is divided into three phases:

- **Getting going**: usually seven sessions either in a group or one-to-one, aimed at introducing the participant to the course
- **My journey**: averaging about 68 sessions of 2½ hours and 11 supported learning sessions. This is designed to understand the 'old me', strengthen the 'new me' and the 'future new me'
- **New me MOT**: delivered by the offender's manager to support the individual through various phases through custody, release and living in the community.

Evaluation of the Kaizen programme is still limited, and as a fairly new programme, will need a substantial number of years to fully evaluate its effect on the recidivism of the offender.

Multi-Agency Public Protection Arrangements (MAPPA)

As the number of people convicted of online sexual offences increases year on year, so does the requirements of their registration, overseen by MAPPA who share information about the registered person. They have three categories of offender: cat 1, all registered sexual offenders (sometimes called a schedule 1 offender); cat 2, violent or other sexual offenders and cat 3, other dangerous offenders. MAPPA have three levels of management: Level 1 is ordinary management between police officers and probation; Level 2 is more multi-agency, perhaps involving social workers or children's guardians, who will have Multi-Agency Public Protection meetings (MAPP); Level 3 are for those deemed the highest risk of causing harm, or whose management is problematic, and will involve a Multi-Agency Protection Panel. The MAPPA system can determine where an offender should live, set exclusion zones within an area, monitor the SHPO and require the offender to report to their Offender Manager, who may be their probation officer, or may be a jigsaw police officer (named after Operation Jigsaw who are part of the public protection team). In extreme cases, they may covertly monitor offenders and/or disclose to the public for their own safety.

The State offers no therapeutic support or treatment for non-convicted individuals who feel out of control of their sexual behaviour, and/or that they may cross the line into committing an offence. Treatment is limited only to those who have been convicted; cure not prevention. Therefore, several external agencies have developed to try and fill the widening gap of need for what is clearly a deluging area of online offending. I will briefly overview these. Although they are not part of the criminal justice system *per se*, knowing what is available for clients can become a valuable part of working with a forensic client.

The Lucy Faithful Foundation (LFF). The LFF is a charity aimed at preventing child sexual abuse. They run an anonymous confidential helpline called Stop It Now, and Shore, a website for teenagers. They run treatment programmes for individuals who have been arrested, cautioned or convicted of online sexual offences. Inform Plus aims to help individuals who view CSAM; Engage Plus focuses on individuals who have engaged in online chat with children. The programmes are group sessions that run for ten sessions of about 2½ hours. For an extra fee, they can be undertaken one-to-one. However, for individuals who have just lost their employment and need to pay for a second home in which to live, the costs of these programmes are out of reach for many. They also run support groups for families, offer training to professionals and have a good research network.

Specialist Treatment Organisation for Perpetrators and Victims of Sexual Offending (StopSO). StopSO is a charity offering nationwide therapeutic help to those who may, or indeed have, committed a sexual offence, or just feel that they are out of control of their own behaviour; as such it has a preventative philosophy. Therapy is conducted on a one-to-one basis with the client either online or face-to-face. The client pays for their therapy directly to their therapist for a fee negotiated between them, not to the organisation. StopSO also have a bursary scheme where some individuals who lack an income can receive up to 12 sessions of therapy free of charge. StopSO therapists have all received specialist training to work in a forensic field. In addition, they offer therapy to the partners and families of offenders, and their direct victims. StopSO also provides supervision and training for their therapist membership to maintain the standards of the work. The therapeutic work that StopSO therapists provide is not just about the working with the offence, but working with the whole individual to enhance their lives and those of their family.

Safer Lives. Safer Lives is based in the West Midlands and Leeds, although offering an online service. It offers individual consultations to lead people into a five-session programme for those over the age of 21 to address online sexual behaviour and offending. They also offer a transition programme for those of 16–21 years of age. As with the LFF, the course is expensive, and increases if the individual is going through the court system, although payments can be made by instalments.

Circles of Support. Circles works with multi-agency support and offers a group of four to six volunteers, family members, probation and the police, to provide a support network toward an individual who has been convicted of harmful sexual behaviour, most commonly after release from prison. They form an outer group, or circle, meeting regularly (usually weekly) to provide support and practical guidance, helping the person take responsibility and to become accountable for their behaviour. Each circle is unique as it is designed to meet the need of the core individual. This support commonly lasts for 12 months, but can be extended if it is considered the person requires additional support. They also offer a short six-month support programme called Circle Reboot for individuals convicted of CSAM offences online.

Conclusion

The criminal justice system (CJS) is being overwhelmed by the number of online offences as a consequence of readily available smart technology. Even the most recent Online Safety Act of 2023, designed to protect children and adults online, is playing catch up with described offences as artificial intelligence (AI) and virtual reality (VR) can take an individual acting out to new highs (or new lows). Individuals getting the knock for online offences are facing up to five years of delays as the system slowly grinds through its process. Getting the knock is a wake-up call for many individuals, who rush off to do the courses and personal therapy offered by the external agencies, and after several years of rehabilitative work, the Criminal Justice System then sends them to prison. Stuck fast in antiquated methods of due process, the development of modern technology, if used appropriately could triage and speed up the whole system if someone dared to say that, as it presents today with these offences, the CJS is broken, is not fit for purpose and needs to be fixed.

References

Andrews, D. A. and Bonta, J. (2013) *The psychology of criminal conduct*, 6th ed. Lexis Nexis/Anderson.

BBC News (2019) Police concerns over rise of 'paedophile hunters'. https://www.bbc.co.uk/news/uk-england-50302912.

Elliott, I & Hambly O. (2023) *Horizon and iHorizon. An uncontrolled before-after study of clinical outcomes*. Ministry of Justice Analytic Series.

Farmer, M., Beech, A. R. & Ward, T. (2012) Assessing desistance in child molesters: a qualitative analysis. *Journal of Interpersonal Violence*, 27, 930–950.

Fouzder, M. (2018) *Offenders 'not getting the support they need' due to decline in pre-sentence reports*. Law Society Gazette. www.lawgazette.co.uk/law/offenders-not-getting-support-they-need-due-to-decline-in-pre-sentence-reports/5066916.article.

Grove, W. M., Zald, D. H., Lebow, B. S., Snitz, B. E. & Nelson, C. (2000) Clinical versus mechanical prediction: A meta-analysis. *Psychological Assessment*, 12, 19–31.

Hart, S. D. & Boer D.P. (2021) Structured Professional Judgement Guidelines for Sexual Violence Risk Assessment. The Sexual Violence Risk-20 (SVR-20) versions 1 and 2 and Risk for Sexual violence Protocol (RSVP). In R. K. Otto & K. S. Douglas (eds) *Handbook of Violence Risk Assessment*. 2nd ed. (pp. 322–358). Routledge.

Horseman, G. (2018) A forensic examination of the technical and legal challenges surrounding the investigation of child abuse on live streaming platforms: A case study on Periscope. *Journal of Information Security and Applications*, 42, 107–117.

Hudson-Allez, G (2004) Threats to psychotherapeutic confidentiality: Can psychotherapists in the UK really offer a confidentiality ethic to their clients? *Psychodynamic Practice*, 10(3), 317–331.

Hudson-Allez, G. (2014) Introduction. In G. Hudson-Allez (ed.) *Sexual Diversity and Sexual Offending. Research, Assessment, and Clinical Treatment in Psychosexual Therapy.* Karnac.

Hudson-Allez, G (2023) *A Trauma-Informed Understanding of Online Offending. Adult Losses from Adolescent Searches.* Routledge.

Lee, Y.-J., Hyeon, J. & Choi, H.-J. (2023) Large language models can share images too! https://arxiv.org/pdf/2310.14804.

McNaughton Nicholls, C. & Webster, S. (2014) *Sex Offender Management and Dynamic Risk: Pilot Evaluation of the Active Risk Management System (ARMS).* Ministry of Justice Analytical Series.

Ministry of Justice (2023) Multi-Agency Public Protection Arrangements (MAPPA) Annual Report 2022/23. https://assets.publishing.service.gov.uk/media/653966ade6c968000daa 9b26/MAPPA_Annual_Report_2023.pdf.

NSPCC (2024) As child abuse image crimes increase, we're calling for Ofcom and tech companies to take action. https://www.nspcc.org.uk/about-us/news-opinion/2024/Child-abuse-image-crimes-increase-calling-ofcom-tech-companies-take-action/.

Ogloff, J. R. P., Cutajar, M. C., Mann, E. & Mullen, P. (2012) Child sexual abuse and subsequent offending and victimisation: A follow-up study. *Trends and Issues in Crime and Criminal Justice,* 440, Australian Institute of Criminology. https://www.aic.gov.au/sites/default/files/2020-05/tandi440.pdf.

Skidmore, M. & Aitkenhead, B. (2022) Turning the Tide on Child Sexual Abuse. The Police Foundation. https://www.police-foundation.org.uk/2022/07/turning-the-tide-on-online-child-sexual-abuse/.

Thornton, D. (2002) Constructing and testing a framework for dynamic risk assessment. *Sexual Abuse: A Journal of Research and Treatment,* 14, 139–153.

Ward, T., Mann, R. E. & Gannon, T.A. (2007). The good lives model of offender rehabilitation: Clinical implications. *Aggression and Violent Behavior,* 12, 87–107.

Webster, S. D., Mann, R. E., Carter, A. J. Long, J. Milner, R. O'Brien, M. D., Wakling, H. & Ray, N. (2006) Inter-rated reliability of dynamic risk assessment with sexual offenders in treatment. *Polygraph,* 34, 171–183.

Zgoba, K. M. & Mitchell, M. M. (2021) The effectiveness of Sex Offender Registration and Notification: A meta-analysis of 25 years of findings. *Journal of Experimental Criminology,* 19, 71–96.

Zilney, L. A. (2021) *Impacts of Sex Crime Laws on the Female Partners of Convicted Offenders. Never Free of Collateral Consequences.* Routledge.

Chapter 6

Sex offenders in numbers and the impact of therapy

Michael Stock

Introduction

Sexual offending has occurred throughout history. Prostitution is called the oldest profession, so sex addiction is not a new phenomenon, although it was not recognised as an addiction until towards the end of the twentieth century, see for example Carnes (2001). The advent of the internet, and in particular broadband, has enabled online sexual activity in the form of sexual communication between adults, and between adults and children. Online pornography is readily accessible and free of charge. Similarly, child sexual abuse material (CSAM) is accessible via websites and through online chat rooms and this has added a whole new dimension to the nature of sexual offending.

Measuring sexual offending has never been easy. Sexual addiction and offending are by nature clandestine activities and most offending pre-internet is estimated to have gone unrecorded. For example, an analysis of sexual offending date carried out jointly by the Ministry of Justice, Home Office and Office for National Statistics (2013) estimated that on an annual basis around 470,000 sexual offences were being committed, whilst sexual offences recorded by the police were around 54,000 annually. Offences such as rape were much more likely to be reported to the police than other offences. This accords with my experience as a therapist who works with offenders, where clients with paraphilias 'unusual sexual behaviours' (Birchard, 2011, 2015) are likely to offend repeatedly with only a small proportion of their offences being recorded by the police. The advent of the internet has, however, made the problem of measuring sexual offending much more difficult. The sheer scale of the internet makes measurement difficult, for example:

> There are over 1.5 billion websites on the world wide web today. Of these, less than 200 million are active. The milestone of 1 billion websites was first reached in September of 2014, as confirmed by **NetCraft** in its October 2014 Web Server Survey and first estimated and announced by **Internet Live Stats** . . . The number had subsequently declined, reverting back to a level below 1 billion (due to the monthly fluctuations in the count of inactive websites) before reaching

DOI: 10.4324/9781003509103-7

again and stabilizing above the 1 billion mark starting in March of 2016. During 2016, the total number of sites has grown significantly, from 900 million in January 2016 to 1.7 billion in December 2016. From 2016 to 2018, the level has hold [sic] pretty much unchanged.

(Internet Live Stats, 2024)

The number of websites today is probably even greater than the numbers in the above quote. In addition, the existence of the dark web, which can only be accessed by specialist browsers such as TOR, a web browser offering complete privacy, makes the detection of illegal activity difficult, and the identity of users of TOR is deliberately hidden. Websites providing illegal material such as CSAM are typically hosted in countries outside the UK and so are not subject to any regulation by UK authorities. The advent of smartphone apps such as Kik and Snapchat have also made it easy to access online material and to message others whilst leaving a minimal audit trail.

Realistically only anecdotal evidence of online illegal behaviour is available. The outcome of sexual offending, be it online or not, can be captured when an offender is arrested and their activity is recorded by the police and the justice system, assuming that they are prosecuted. But this will be only a small proportion of total offending behaviour. The approach in this chapter is to first give a brief description of the scale of online offending, then to look at estimated offending in the UK using published official sources. The characteristics of offenders are then examined in more detail and these are then compared with the StopSO clients who filled in questionnaires. Finally, there is an analysis of the questionnaire data, with particular emphasis on the change reported by clients after 12 weeks of therapy with a StopSO registered therapist.

Online offending

The Internet Watch Foundation is a charity that investigates and seeks to have removed websites containing CSAM:

The IWF has just marked 25 years as a charity dealing with Child Sexual Abuse Material (CSAM) Online. Over that period, we have assessed 1.8 million reports and actioned 970,000 reports for removal. Each of these reports can contain from one to thousands of individual images, meaning we have removed millions of child sexual abuse images and videos from the internet in the past 25 years.

In 2021, we investigated more reports of suspected child sexual abuse imagery than the entire first 15 years we were in existence. In the period 1996–2011 we assessed 335,558 reports and in 2021, we investigated 361,000 reports including from members of the public and our analysts own proactive searches. Of these reports, the IWF confirmed 252,000 reports as containing Child Sexual

Abuse Material and the number of reports we actioned for removal in 2021, had increased by 64% on 2020's figures. We have also witnessed over the past decade a worrying increase in the number of girls appearing in these images. Ten years ago, girls appeared in 67% of the imagery we removed, in 2021, it was 97%.

(Internet Watch Foundation, 2022

Another concerning trend seen in the IWF data has been the rise in what is now called 'self-generated' indecent images of children. The imagery has been produced by children themselves via webcam and then uploaded, shared, or streamed online. These images are then harvested from their original upload location in a process known as 'capping' and then shared on dedicated child sexual abuse websites. Since 2019 there has been a 374% rise in self-generated imagery, with the 11–13 age range of young girls appearing the most. In the first quarter of 2022, the IWF identified that the children in these images were getting younger, with 20,000 incidents identified amongst **7–10-year-olds** (IWF, 2022).

The growth in activity is enormous and underlines the scale of CSAM on the internet. There is also mention of self-generated material. A new development that is just starting to have an impact is the use of artificial intelligence (AI) to produce CSAM and other illegal material. At the 2023 StopSO conference, a representative of CEOP (Child Exploitation and Online Protection), a command of the National Crime Agency (NCA), predicted that AI would lead to a further significant increase in CSAM and make it even more difficult to detect (Marsh, 2023).

In their annual report for 2022 (Internet Watch Foundation, 2023) the IWF reports investigating 375,200 websites in 2022, an increase of 4% since 2021 and notes the proportion of category A CSAM images detected (penetration, sexual activity with an animal, sadism) has increased from 17% to 20% between 2020 and 2022, category B images (non-penetrative sexual activity) have increased from 16% to 26%, whilst category C (other indecent images not falling in categories A or B) have declined from 68% to 54%. The predominant ages of the children depicted in the CSAM are seven to ten years and 11 to 13 years across all three categories. Of these images, 73% are of girls, 22% are of boys and the remainder (6%) are either both or other (percentages add to over 100% because of rounding). The most common types of activity shown were non-penetrative sex (33%), penetration (25%), sexual posing with nudity (17%) and masturbation (11%).

The scale of sexual offending in the UK

In this section sexual offending statistics are drawn from three key sources: offenders processed by the criminal justice system, police records of arrests and investigations and the Crime Survey for England and Wales (CSEW). The first two sources are taken from administrative records and only deal with reported crimes. The latter source differs from the first because it is based on a statistical sample of adults in England and Wales, which are asked in face-to-face interviews about their experience of crime in the past 12 months, whether reported to the police or not, and it also asks them for their lifetime experience of being a victim of crime. It will be less precise than the administrative sources since it is sample-based and depends upon respondents accurately describing their experience, but it provides a way of estimating the overall level of sexual offending in the UK.

Table 6.1 summarises the experience of sexual crime by sex of victim. Over one quarter of women report being a victim of a sexual crime during their lifetime, compared to 6.1% for men. Similarly the rates in the last year are very different with 3.2% of women and 0.9% of men reporting an incident. Unwanted sexual touching (21%) and indecent exposure (11.6%) are high figures for women.

Table 6.2 shows police recorded sexual offences over time. For various reasons the changes over time should be treated with caution since recording methods have changed and more recently more crimes have been reported following encouragement by the police to do so. Nevertheless, there have been sustained increases in all categories, but whilst overall reported sexual offences have increased 340%, rape (569%) and sexual activity with minors have increased much more (675%), probably reflecting better reporting in the case of rape and an increase in internet offences.

Sex offenders are almost exclusively male (99%) compared to 85% of all offenders (January–March 2022). In that period 24% of all offenders had reoffended (Ministry of Justice, 2024). This compares with sex offenders where only 13% were reoffenders. Typically, around 80% of sex offenders in the period 2005–2011 had no previous conviction and this was fairly stable across all the different types of offence (rape, sexual assault, sexual activity with a minor, other) (Ministry of Justice, 2013).

The proportion of sex offenders in the prison population rose between 2005 and 2011. In 2011, there were 10,935 prisoners in custody for sexual offences, an increase of 57% since 2005. The proportion of sex offenders in prison rose from 9% in 2005 to 14% of the overall prison population by 2011. As of 31 March 2020 there were 12,774 prisoners serving sentences for sexual offences, which represented 18% of the sentenced prison population. This was a slight decline since 2018 (Ministry of Justice, 2021).

Characteristics and behaviour of StopSO clients

StopSO (Specialist Treatment Organisation for Perpetrators and Survivors of Sexual Offending) receives enquiries from actual or potential sex offenders who are seeking one-to-one therapy. StopSO then refers them to one of the therapists registered with them, normally on the basis of geographical proximity to maximise the option for face-to-face rather than online therapy. StopSO therapists must have a minimum level of training set by StopSO. Once a referral has been made and accepted and the enquirer has become a client of a StopSO therapist then StopSO sends a pre-therapy evaluation form to the client to be completed at the start of

Table 6.1 Likelihood of being a victim of a sexual crime

	Percentage of men who were victims once or more since the age of 16	Percentage of women who were victims once or more since the age of 16	Percentage of men who were victims once or more in the last year	Percentage of women who were victims once or more in the last year
Sexual assault by rape or penetration including attempts	6.1	26.5	0.9	3.2
Sexual assault by rape or penetration excluding attempts	0.8	8.6	0.1	0.8
Rape including attempts	0.5	7.0	0.1	0.4
Rape excluding attempts	0.6	7.5	0.1	0.5
Assault by penetration including attempts	0.4	6.1	0.0	0.3
Assault by penetration excluding attempts	0.5	6.3	0.1	0.6
Indecent exposure or unwanted sexual touching	0.3	4.6	0.1	0.2
Indecent exposure	5.8	25.4	0.8	2.9
Unwanted sexual touching	1.6	11.6	0.2	0.8
Any sexual assault (including attempts) by a partner	5.0	21.0	0.7	2.3
Sexual assault by rape or penetration (including attempts) by a partner	1.0	7.9	0.1	0.4
Indecent exposure or unwanted sexual touching by a partner	0.2	4.8	0.1	0.2
Indecent exposure by a partner	0.9	7.0	0.1	0.3
Unwanted sexual touching by a partner	0.2	0.9	[c]	[c]
Any sexual assault (including attempts) by a family member	0.9	6.9	0.1	0.3
Sexual assault by rape or penetration (including attempts) by a family member	0.2	2.4	[c]	0.1
Indecent exposure or unwanted sexual touching by a family member	0.2	2.0	[c]	0.0
Indecent exposure by a family member	0.1	0.7	[c]	[c]
Unwanted sexual touching by a family member	0.1	1.6	[c]	0.0

Source: Crime Survey for England and Wales. Office for National Statistics(reproduced with permission).

Notes: subcategory percentages may exceed total because respondent appears in more than one subcategory.

[c] indicates numbers too small to publish.

Table 6.2 Police recorded sexual offences England and Wales

	Total rape	Total sexual assault	Total sexual activity with minors	Total other sexual offences	Total sexual offences
2003	12,295	29,407	3,615	11,335	56,652
2004	13,272	31,350	4,110	11,680	60,412
2005	14,013	28,176	4,890	13,845	60,924
2006	14,443	26,189	5,491	14,164	60,287
2007	13,774	24,158	5,275	12,835	56,042
2008	12,673	23,198	5,141	11,154	52,166
2009	13,096	22,063	5,140	9,886	50,185
2010	15,074	22,103	5,809	10,020	53,006
2011	15,892	23,055	5,808	9,185	53,940
2012	16,038	22,057	5,779	8,886	52,760
2013	16,374	22,365	6,641	8,219	53,599
2014	20,751	26,115	8,773	8,593	64,232
2015	29,420	34,940	13,388	10,828	88,576
2016	36,334	41,608	17,483	11,806	107,231
2017	42,063	46,342	21,278	13,311	122,994
2018	55,004	56,057	23,563	18,117	152,741
2019	59,921	59,509	25,126	19,752	164,308
2020	59,104	58,796	24,536	20,808	163,244
2021	55,652	49,844	22,260	20,079	147,835
2022	69,905	75,023	24,419	24,219	193,566

Source: Office for National Statistics (reproduced with permission).

therapy and returned directly to StopSO. Clients are given a strong guarantee that their answers will be treated as confidential and once the data are coded, it is impossible to identify individual clients. A mid-therapy evaluation form is then sent after 12 weeks to enable an assessment of the progress and impact of therapy. The analysis in this section focuses first on the pre-evaluation forms to provide information on the characteristics of clients, before looking at how the client's behaviour and feelings have changed as a result of therapy, by comparing some of the answers from the pre-evaluation forms with the mid-evaluation form answers. The term StopSO client is used for simplicity but strictly the enquirers become clients of the individual therapists rather than StopSO.

The StopSO evaluation forms returned are not based on a statistical sample of StopSO clients and so may not be representative of StopSO clients as a whole, but the number of pre-evaluation forms that have been returned makes it reasonable to assume that they are fairly representative of StopSO clients. The number of mid-evaluation forms is much lower and therefore is less likely to be representative.

Some StopSO clients had not had any involvement with the police or the legal system, around 15% of those returning pre-evaluation forms, and had contacted StopSO because they were troubled by their fantasies. They have not been separated out since the numbers on the mid-evaluation forms would have been too small to allow analysis.

StopSO clients are almost all male: 93% reported being male, 5% did not state their sex and the other 2% reported being trans or other. For the purposes of comparison StopSO clients are compared to the male population in England and Wales. The age of clients is shown in Table 6.3.

The population percentages have been calculated from population date published by the Office for National Statistics and relate to 2021. The 26–35 and 36–45 age groups are heavily over represented in the StopSO client data compared to the population, 49% compared to 29%, whereas those aged 66 or over comprise only 8% of the StopSO clients compared with 23% in the population.

The ethnicity of StopSO clients is shown in Table 6.4.

For comparison 82% of men identified as white in the census. All non-white ethnic groups are under-represented in the StopSO data.

The sexual orientation of StopSO clients is shown in Table 6.5.

Three quarters of clients report as heterosexual, the only other significant groups being bisexual (11%) and gay (8%). Whilst there are no definitive statistics available on the proportion of men who identify as gay, 8% is higher than estimates based on survey data, for example the National Survey of Sexual Attitudes

Table 6.3 Age of StopSO clients

Age of StopSO Clients			% Population
16–18	9	2%	4%
19–25	76	14%	10%
26–35	133	25%	15%
36–45	128	24%	14%
45–55	83	15%	17%
56–65	61	11%	17%
66–75	33	6%	13%
75+	9	2%	10%
ns	10	2%	
Total	542	100%	100%

Source: StopSO evaluation forms. Office for National Statistics (reproduced with permission).

Table 6.4 Ethnicity of StopSO clients

White	493	91%
Black	4	1%
Asian	12	2%
Other	18	3%
Other minority ethnic	1%	1%
Not specified	9	2%
Total	542	100%

Source: StopSO Evaluation Forms (reproduced with permission).

Table 6.5 Sexual orientation of StopSO clients

Heterosexual	403	74%
Gay	44	8%
Trans	0	0%
Lesbian	1	0%
Bisexual	57	11%
Asexual	6	1%
Queer	4	1%
Other	17	3%
Not stated	10	2%
Total	542	100%

Source: StopSO Evaluation Forms (reproduced with permission).

Table 6.6 What difficulties have you experienced that led you to choose a StopSO therapist?

You have been charged and are facing criminal proceedings	78	14%
The police have been involved but you have not been charged yet	292	54%
You have been scared about your sexual fantasies but have no police involvement	81	15%
You have been sentenced after committing a sexual offence	39	7%
Multiple answers	35	6%
Not stated	17	3%
Total	542	100%

Source: StopSO Evaluation Forms (reproduced with permission).

and Lifestyles (Natsal), which gathers data on sexual behaviour and attitudes in Britain estimated that between 2010 and 2012, 1.5% of men identified as gay or homosexual.

The reasons clients gave for contacting StopSO are shown in Table 6.6.

The largest group had been involved with the police but had not yet been charged, whilst 21% have been charged or sentenced for committing a sexual offence. This confirms that most clients do not approach StopSO until they have been involved with the police or the legal system.

Table 6.7 reports on viewing of illegal child images.

Overall, of those who stated their activity, 53% mentioned viewing images, but the way the data were collected was ambiguous and some clients may have only responded to only one category, for example collecting images implies viewing them. Collecting was mentioned by 28% and sharing by 20%, but it should be noted that 33% did not state their activity, possibly because they were not able to state in the questionnaire that they had not viewed images but had committed other offences. So, the data should be treated with caution since not stated may mean the question was not applicable. Overall, however, it seems reasonable to conclude that a clear majority of StopSO clients had viewed illegal images, with some collecting or sharing them.

Table 6.7 Viewing collecting and sharing illegal images of children

Have you been viewing Illegal images?	148	27%
Have you been collecting illegal images?	8	1%
Have you been viewing Illegal images and collecting illegal images?	88	16%
Have you been viewing Illegal images and have you been sharing illegal images?	51	9%
Have you been viewing Illegal images, sharing illegal images and collecting illegal images?	60	11%
Other	7	1%
Not stated	180	33%
Total	542	100%

Source: StopSO Evaluation Forms (reproduced with permission).

Table 6.8 Ages of children viewed

0–4	0	0%
5–9	0	0%
9–12	3	3%
5–17	9	9%
9–17	22	21%
13–17	24	23%

Source: StopSO Evaluation Forms (reproduced with permission).

The ages of children viewed are shown in Table 6.8.

Unfortunately, the evaluation form allowed free format answers or concatenated answers, and so it is not possible to provide a quantitative analysis of the answers. However, based on an analysis of a subset of answers it seems that the child victim age groups 5–17, 9–17 and 13–17 are common. None of the responses mentioned children below nine. The conclusion can be drawn that children approaching pubescence and early post-pubescent children are the main focus of illegal image viewing. Both girls and boys were viewed, but girls are mentioned more often than boys. When asked had they tried to contact the children whose images they had viewed, 15% said yes, 65% said no, with the remaining 19% not giving an answer.

Table 6.9 shows what clients watched online. Almost half of clients did not provide an answer and the only significant number of responses related to voyeurism (34%).

Responses to other questions had high levels of non-response but the responses show that 27% of clients had posted sexual images of themselves online; only 3% had posted sexually explicit images of a current or former partner; 4% had placed a camera without someone's knowledge; 4% had taken photographs of children; 8% had touched an adult inappropriately and 6% had touched a child, but 85% did not answer the question on touching a child, although presumably the answer was no; 4% had made someone do something sexual they did not want to.

Table 6.9 Internet viewing of StopSO clients

Bestiality	16	4%
Voyeurism	153	34%
Sexual violence against women	12	3%
Sexual violence against all of these	10	2%
Voyeurism and sexual violence against women	12	3%
Voyeurism and bestiality	24	5%
Voyeurism, bestiality and sexual violence against women	15	3%
Other combinations	20	4%
Not stated	190	42%
Total	452	100

Source: StopSO Evaluation Forms (reproduced with permission).

Table 6.10 How strongly do you feel sexual attraction to different subjects

	0	1 to 5	6 to 10	Not stated	Total
Men	299	148	75	20	542
	55%	27%	14%	4%	100%
Women	41	62	426	13	542
	8%	11%	79%	2%	100%
Teenage boys	394	80	43	25	542
	73%	15%	8%	5%	100%
Teenage girls	195	146	176	25	542
	36%	27%	32%	5%	100%
Younger boys	428	60	27	27	542
	79%	11%	5%	5%	100%
Younger girls	341	117	60	24	542
	63%	22%	11%	4%	100%
Toddlers	475	33	10	24	542
	88%	6%	2%	4%	100%
Babies	499	16	3	24	542
	92%	3%	1%	4%	100%
Animals	473	36	10	23	542
	87%	7%	2%	4%	100%

Source StopSO Evaluation Forms (reproduced with permission).

A high proportion (82%) of clients said that they watched pornography but the data regarding the amount watched was too sparse to analyse formally. Reported amounts varied from a few hours a week up to 25 hours or more. Similarly, the format of responses on the age when the client first saw pornography were difficult to analyse but a sample analysis suggests that 40% of clients saw pornography before the age of ten, a further 45% saw it before the age of 15 and only 15% of clients first saw pornography after the age of 15.

Table 6.10 reports the strength of sexual attraction that clients felt.

Women created the strongest response with 79% of clients scored in the range 6–10, whilst 59% reported an attraction to teenage girls (27% scored 1–5 and

32% 6–10) and 33% to younger girls (22% and 11%). Clients felt a lower attraction to men; 41% (27% and 14 %) compared to women (79% 6–10), lower attraction to teenage boys, 23% compared with 59% and lower attraction to younger boys, 16% compared to 33%. Clients reported a low attraction to toddlers, babies and animals.

Table 6.11 reports on masturbation fantasies. Voyeurism or dogging is the most common at 39% (26% and 13%); next comes children not known to the client with 31% of clients responding (20% and 11%); very similar is being watched whilst having sex at 27% (19% and 8%); then rape in fantasy 26% (20% and 6%). Some 12% of clients masturbated to a fantasy of hurting someone and 7% to raping someone in real life, whilst 3% masturbated to the thought of killing someone. Whilst lower than responses to other masturbatory fantasies these figures regarding hurting someone are nevertheless still concerning.

Table 6.12 looks at the impact on various aspects of the client's life. High impacts are reported for all areas, the exception being impact on the client's children, but clients were not able to specify that they had no children, so the 47% reporting no impact probably includes a significant number of clients without children. Three

Table 6.11 When you masturbate do you think about:

	0	1–5	6–10	Not stated	Total
Children known to you	453	49	19	21	542
	84%	9%	4%	4%	100%
Children not known to you	356	106	62	18	542
	66%	20%	11%	3%	100%
Animals	473	40	9	20	542
	87%	7%	2%	4%	100%
Rape in fantasy	383	106	35	18	542
	71%	20%	6%	3%	100%
Rape in real life	482	29	11	20	542
	89%	5%	2%	4%	100%
Hurting someone	455	52	13	22	542
	84%	10%	2%	4%	100%
Killing someone	504	14	2	22	542
	93%	3%	0%	4%	100%
Exposing yourself	444	50	28	20	542
	82%	9%	5%	4%	100%
Watched whilst having sex	371	104	45	22	542
	68%	19%	8%	4%	100%
Voyeurism or dogging	302	142	73	25	542
	56%	26%	13%	5%	100%
Rubbing against strangers	489	24	7	22	542
	90%	4%	1%	4%	100%
Secretly taking pictures	468	36	14	24	542
	86%	7%	3%	4%	100%

Source: StopSO Evaluation Forms (reproduced with permission).

Table 6.12 What has been the impact on your:

	0	1–5	6–10	Not stated	Total
Job	105	124	294	19	542
	19%	23%	54%	4%	100%
Homelife	141	115	405	12	542
	26%	21%	75%	2%	100%
Relationship with partner	109	91	405	44	542
	20%	17%	75%	8%	100%
Your sex life	109	91	298	44	542
	20%	17%	55%	8%	100%
Your children	256	38	155	93	542
	47%	7%	29%	17%	100%
Family members	86	116	313	27	542
	16%	21%	58%	5%	100%
Finances	141	166	207	28	542
	26%	31%	38%	5%	100%
Friends and social life	64	134	325	64	542
	12%	25%	60%	12%	100%

Source: StopSO Evaluation Forms (reproduced with permission).

Table 6.13 Importance of sex and pornography

	0	1 to 5	6 to 10	Not stated	Total
Importance of sex in your life	53	218	259	12	542
	10%	40%	48%	2%	100%
Importance of pornography	111	255	165	11	542
	20%	47%	30%	2%	100%

Source: StopSO Evaluation Forms (reproduced with permission).

quarters reported a high impact (scoring 6–10) on their relationship with their partner and their homelife, with 60% reporting a high impact on friends and social life and 58% for family members.

Table 6.13 shows the importance of sex and pornography in the lives of clients with 40% scoring 1–5 for the importance of sex and 48 % scoring 6–10. For pornography 47% scored 1–5 and 30% 6–10.

Table 6.14 shows levels of distress and suicidal thoughts and the motivation to change, the specific question wording, which is somewhat lengthy for a table, was 'How determined are you to change your sexual behaviour?'. Clients reported very high levels of distress with only 1% reporting no distress (0) and 78% reporting high distress. Whilst a little lower, the reports of suicidal feelings are still high with 81% (42% and 39%) reporting suicidal feelings. The motivation to change was also very high with 92% responding in the 6–10 range and of these 497 responses 381 were 10.

Table 6.14 Level of distress and motivation to change

	0	1–5	6–10	Not stated	Total
How distressed are you feeling	7	104	422	9	542
	1%	19%	78%	2%	100%
Have you been feeling suicidal	96	226	211	96	542
	18%	42%	39%	18%	100%
Motivation to change	14	17	497	14	542
	3%	3%	92%	3%	100%

Source: StopSO Evaluation Forms (reproduced with permission).

Table 6.15 Number of sessions of therapy to date

less than 5	0
5 to 10	1
10 to 15	25
15 to 20	3
20 or more	5
not stated	1
Total	35

Source: StopSO Evaluation Forms (reproduced with permission).

Turning to the mid-evaluation forms only 35 were returned but this is sufficient to draw some tentative conclusions, particularly as the changes from the pre-evaluation forms is marked. Table 6.15 shows the number of therapy sessions completed at the point the mid-evaluation form was returned by the client. Most had completed between ten and 15 and none less than five which is consistent with sending the forms out after 12 weeks from the acceptance of the referral by the therapist.

Of some concern is that of the 35 clients, 27 reported still watching pornography, with only six saying no with two not stated.

The extent of change between the two sets of forms is shown in Table 6.16.

A level of distress is still reported by 92% of clients at mid-evaluation but the proportion reporting in the 6–10 range has declined from 78% to 46%. Even though the mid-evaluation analysis is based on only 35 forms this is still a significant change. Similarly, the level of suicidal thoughts is still high but the proportion in the 6–10 range has reduced from 39% to 17%. The importance of sex is only slightly reduced, but perhaps of concern is that 71% of clients still report that pornography is important to them with 14% in the higher range.

The textual responses to the question on the mid-evaluation forms almost all mention how helpful the therapy has been to date. This is in line with the lower reports of distress and suicidal thoughts. Clients also frequently mention how therapy

Table 6.16 Change between pre- and mid-evaluation forms

Your feelings					
Distress			*Suicidal thoughts*		
	Pre	*Mid*		*Pre*	*Mid*
0	1%	6%	0	18%	20%
1–5	19%	46%	1–5	42%	60%
6–10	78%	46%	6–10	39%	17%
Not Stated	2%	3%	Not Stated	2%	3%
Total	100%	100%	Total	100%	100%
Importance of Sex			*Importance of Pornography*		
	Pre	*Mid*		*Pre*	*Mid*
0	10%	3%	0	20%	26%
1–5	40%	57%	1–5	64%	57%
6–10	48%	37%	6–10	16%	14%
Not Stated	2%	3%	Not Stated	0%	3%
Total	100%	100%		100%	100%

Source: StopSO Evaluation Forms (reproduced with permission).

has helped them understand why they offended and how issues from their past had been a factor in their offending. They also mentioned developing strategies to avoid re-offending and being able to more open with partners. Some had gained a better understanding of the legal process.

Data from the Independent Enquiry into Child Sexual Abuse

Finally, this section reports some of the data collected by the Independent Inquiry into Child Sex Abuse (IICSA) (IICSA, 2022a). As part of this inquiry nearly 6,000 people shared their experience of sexual abuse and consented to their responses being published as statistical tables. The data are contained in the IICSA data compendium (IICSA, 2022b). As with the StopSO data the responses were not based on a random sample and so may not be typical of all survivors of sexual abuse. The data relate mostly to contact offences and as such differ from the StopSO data, where online offending without contact predominates. Nevertheless, the IICSA data demonstrates the profound impact that child sex abuse has and is included here to put the responses of StopSO clients into context.

Table 6.17 shows the age at which the sexual abuse started (the format used by IICSA of putting percentages first has been retained to allow comparison with the source document). The predominant age ranges are 4–7 and 8–11, somewhat

Table 6.17 Age at which sexual abuse started

0–3 years old	12%	686
4–7 years old	35%	1,936
8–11 years old	32%	1,745
12–15 years old	18%	1,006
16–17 years old	2%	116
Total		5,489

Source: IICSA (reproduced with permission).

Table 6.18 Sexual abuse experienced

Involving penetration	50%	2,920
Sexual touching	57%	3,314
Other contact abuse	44%	2,601
Violations of privacy	19%	1,107
Exposing children to adult sexuality	22%	1,298
Sexual grooming	24%	1,395
Exploitation	7%	431
Other types	2%	97
Total		5,862

Source: IICSA (reproduced with permission).

Note: Respondents could choose multiple categories.

younger than the age groups that StopSO clients reported, see Table 6.8, where the predominant range was 9–17.

Table 6.18 shows the type of abuse experienced. Participants were able to specify more than one type so the individual categories add to more than the total participants. As mentioned above, the participants reported on a large number of contact offences, whilst StopSO clients reported high levels of viewing illegal images, see Table 6.7. Some StopSO clients have committed contact offences, but the data did not allow this to be identified. Participants reported that 47% of abuse was perpetrated by a family member and 42% of abuse happened in the family home.

Table 6.19 shows the impact of the sexual abuse experienced by participants. As with Table 6.18 participants were able to specify more than one category. The impact on mental health they reported is strikingly high.

Table 6.20 shows the pattern of reporting sexual abuse. Two thirds of survivors did not report the abuse at the time and some kept the abuse secret after it ended. Some 9% of participants were disclosing sexual abuse for the first time.

Table 6.19 Impacts of sexual abuse mentioned by participants

	Female		Male		All participants	
Physical health	1,433	35%	550	32%	1,997	34%
Mental health	3,641	90%	1,462	85%	5,143	88%
Sexual behaviour	1,322	33%	479	28%	1,812	31%
Criminal behaviour	188	5%	323	19%	513	9%
School/Employment	1,635	40%	743	43%	2,389	41%
Relationships	2,281	56%	830	48%	3,132	53%
Total	4,065		1,716		5,862	

Source: IICSA (reproduced with permission).

Note: Respondents could choose multiple categories.

Table 6.20 Told someone about the sexual abuse

At the time the abuse was happening			After the abuse ended		
Yes	27%	1,420	Yes	81%	3,934
No	67%	3,575	No	16%	759
Some episodes reported	7%	363	Some episodes reported	4%	173
Total	100%	5,358	Total	100%	4,866

Source: IICSA (reproduced with permission).

Note: Not all respondents answered this question.

Conclusion

Sexual offences involving children recorded in UK official statistics have grown at twice the rate of total sexual offences in the 20 years to 2022. This reflects the rapid expansion of the high speed internet since it was introduced in the UK in 2000.Before the internet sexual offending involved contact between people but the internet has facilitated widespread viewing of pornography and given rise to a new classes of sexual offence involving viewing illegal sexual images of children; online grooming of children; and arranging to have sexual contact with children. Survey evidence confirms that the actual level of sexual offending is much higher than the numbers reported in official statistics. Measuring online offending in the UK is extremely difficult, because of the huge number of sexual content websites available, the fact that the illegal ones are hosted in other countries outside the jurisdiction of the UK police and the existence of tools that allow people to hide their identities. The StopSO evaluation forms give a detailed picture of the type of clients who approach them for help. They are all men, younger than the general population, and around three quarters have been involved with the police and may have been charged or even sentenced before they seek help from StopSO. They generally did not try to contact children they may have had contact with online. The ages of the children in illegal images were typically 9–17 with some as young as five. They looked at voyeurism and masturbated to fantasies of voyeurism and dogging, images of children not known to them and fantasises of being watched whilst having sex and rape. They report high levels of distress and suicidal thoughts and high impact on their relationship with their partner, family, friends, finances and employment. They were strongly motivated to change and the mid-evaluation forms showed that they found therapy helpful, they were focussing on minimising the risk of re-offending and their distress and suicidal thoughts had reduced markedly.

References

Birchard, T. (2011) Sexual Addiction and the Paraphilias. *Sexual Addiction and Compulsivity* 18(3), 157–187.

Birchard, T. (2015) *CBT for Compulsive Sexual Behaviour. A Guide for Professionals.* Routledge.

Carnes, P. (2001) *Out of the Shadows: Understanding Sexual Addiction.* 3rd ed. Hazelden.

Independent Inquiry into Child Sex Abuse (2022a) The Report of the Independent Inquiry into Child Sexual Abuse. www.iicsa.org.uk/final-report.html.

Independent Inquiry into Child Sex Abuse (2022b) The Report of the Independent Inquiry into Child Sexual Abuse – Data Compendium. https://www.iicsa.org.uk/document/report-independent-inquiry-child-sexual-abuse-data-compendium.html.

Internet Live Stats (2024) https://www.internetlivestats.com/total-number-of-websites/.

Internet Watch Foundation (2022) IWF Response to Ofcom Call for Evidence First Phase of online Safety Consultation September 2022. https://www.iwf.org.uk/policy-work/uk-policy/.

Internet Watch Foundation (2023) Annual Report 2022. https://annualreport2022.iwf.org.uk/wp-content/uploads/2023/04/IWF-Annual-Report-2022_FINAL.pdf.

Marsh, A. (2023) Offender Misuse of emerging new technologies. A law enforcement perspective. Paper presented at the StopSO conference, Birmingham, 29 September 2023.

Ministry of Justice, Home Office & the Office for National Statistics (2013) An Overview of Sexual Offending in England and Wales. https://www.gov.uk/government/statistics/an-overview-of-sexual-offending-in-england-and-wales.

Ministry of Justice (2016) Story of the Prison Population 1993 to 2016. https://www.gov.uk/government/statistics/story-of-the-prison-population-1993-to-2016.

Ministry of Justice (2021) Offender management statistics quarterly: October to December 2019 and annual 2019. https://www.gov.uk/government/statistics/offender-management-statistics-quarterly-october-to-december-2019/offender-management-statistics-quarterly-october-to-december-2019-and-annual-2019.

Ministry of Justice, (2024) Proven Reoffending Tables (3 monthly) January to March 2022. https://www.gov.uk/government/statistics/proven-reoffending-statistics-january-to-march-2022 .

Office for National Statistics (2023a) Sexual Offences Prevalence and Trends England and Wales Year Ending March 2022. https://www.ons.gov.uk/peoplepopulationandcommunity/crimeandjustice/articles/sexualoffencesprevalenceandtrendsenglandandwales/yearendingmarch2022.

Office for National Statistics (2023b) Sexual Offences Prevalence and victim Characteristics England and Wales year Ending March 2022. https://www.ons.gov.uk/peoplepopulation andcommunity/crimeandjustice/datasets/sexualoffencesprevalenceandvictimcharacteris ticsenglandandwales.

Office for National Statistics (2024) ONS Statistical bulletin, Crime in England and Wales, year ending September 2023. https://www.ons.gov.uk/peoplepopulationandcommunity/ crimeandjustice/datasets/crimeinenglandandwalesannualsupplementarytables.

Section 2

Working with the variety of presentations

Not a one-size-fits-all approach

Chapter 7

The therapeutic journey

Working with fear, loss, and shame

Ian Richards

Introduction: the knock

'The knock' is a term used to describe the moment, generally early in the morning, that a small group of police officers, sometimes in plain clothing, arrive on the doorstep of an individual, usually a male, and knock loudly on the door of someone they believe has committed a sexual offence, usually online. This event can bring fear into the whole household and destroy the lives of many in it. The accused is often shell-shocked after being woken up to heavy banging on his front door. Dogs are barking, children are rubbing their eyes, and their partner is wondering what the hell is happening. It is a moment never to be forgotten by the whole family, with a possible wait of anything up to two and a half years of living in secrecy, anxiety, and loss.

Initially, the alleged offender will be stunned, suffering from anxiety and often contemplating suicide. If they have children under the age of 18, they will generally be ordered to move out of their home, with their marriage/partnership either broken or hanging by a thread. Most certainly, his employment will either be at risk or perhaps lost. Family and friends often remove themselves from their relationship, sometimes banishing them.

Seeking therapy

This work can be complex, often dealing with childhood trauma, addiction, and always grief. It will be exploring the loss of their home, their wife/partner, their children, their family, friends, and always their dignity and respect. When the therapist speaks to them for the first time, often on the telephone, they are usually scared and feel vulnerable. Meeting them in their initial session, often via Zoom, they can be subdued, quiet, and avoid eye contact. It is important to remember that they may zone out while contracting with them. I will ask them what they are looking to gain from therapy and the answer is often the same, the need to understand what happened.

DOI: 10.4324/9781003509103-9

Face-to-face sessions

If you agree to see your client face-to-face in a counselling practice venue you should always consider the following:

1. Never leave the client alone in a waiting room while you are not there, you never know if a child (under 18) will enter the practice. If this happens, he will be in breach of any order made against him, for example, his bail conditions, Sexual Risk Order (SRO), and Sexual Harm Prevention Order (SHPO).
2. Make sure you are there at least 15 minutes early and inform the client to wait outside until you call him.
3. Be there to greet him at the entrance.
4. If he wishes to use the toilet, check that it is available and wait for him outside.
5. Always escort the client out of the building when therapy has ended.
6. Itemise all of the above into your contract agreement.

The therapist must be aware of their biases and judgements. Establishing a trusting and empathic safe place for their client is crucial as this forms the foundation of their therapeutic relationship (Erskine, 2023, p.141). They will be seeking help from us, a stranger, from whom they hope to gain some understanding of their actions. Their world has crashed around them, and they will feel lost, remorseful, and ashamed. Ask phenomenological questions and be curious about their experience of the nature of their offending. Overall, the most important thing a therapist must do in this work is to create a supportive and collaborative environment where clients feel valued, understood, and empowered.

'Jack'

The following is the case study of Jack, which is in three parts. He is a fictional character, and I would like you to notice what is happening to you while reading the unfolding story while Jack is in therapy. Jack's therapist is named David.

Jack's story Part 1: Session 1

David contracts with Jack before asking him what he wishes to gain from therapy. Jack looks at the therapist and then drops his gaze to the floor. He says nothing and then they enter a minute or two of silence.

David: Jack, I am wondering if it is difficult for you to be here today. *He acknowledges the therapist by nodding his head but still, he says nothing. The therapist waits a few seconds before reminding him of what he stated when contracting.*

David:	Jack, as I said, this is a safe place for you, and I am happy to sit with you in silence if that is what you would prefer.
Jack:	As of this morning, I have no home, and I must move back to my parents as my wife has said it's over between us.
David:	I am sorry to hear this Jack. I can't imagine how devastating this is for you on top of what's happened. *Jack nods his head in agreement.*
Jack:	We had just moved into our home three weeks ago. It was lovely and it was what I had always wanted – I felt that I had achieved something at last.
David:	You say that 'you achieved something at last' Jack, that seems like you are being harsh on yourself.
Jack:	That's because it's true, I have never amounted to anything, and now this. I mean wtf . . . *he says while shaking his head.*
David:	Yes, this must be a challenging time for you.
Jack:	He looks up towards the therapist and says, what makes you want to work with people like me?
David:	'People like you?' . . . because I like what I do, and I appreciate the client inviting me into their world and allowing me to engage with them in their time of dismay.
Jack:	I feel like a complete monster.
David:	And of course, you are not. You have made a mistake and made some bad decisions, but that doesn't make you a monster. *In this first part, Jack struggled to engage in eye contact with his therapist. This would seemingly highlight his feelings of guilt and shame. David allowed him the space to be vulnerable while therapeutically offering him a place of safety.*

In the past, it was quite normal in sexual offender programmes for the offender to provide a detailed description of their offending early in their therapy. This negative attrition would often lead to negative consequences and a higher fallout rate of individuals in therapy. Ward, Hudson, and Keenan (1998) argued that focusing on an offender's necessary risk factors was only a basic aim and not necessarily sufficient to rehabilitate an offender. I have had many clients who have stated that they feel constantly judged. 'It doesn't matter who I look at, I wonder if they know what I have done', one client stated. 'Can they see through my eyes into the monster that I am?', another asked me. 'I can't speak to my in-laws, even though my wife has said they are worried about me,' another client remarked. 'When I look in the mirror, I see this despicable human being that is not worthy of a life and any future happiness', another man said while sobbing.

The Good Life Model (GLM) (Ward & Stewart, 2003) is a strength-based approach which focuses on promoting the strengths of a sex offender while in rehabilitation. It helps the offender to understand their behaviour and develop more positive relational needs by focusing on their values. The GLM focuses on the individual's strengths and helps them find healthier ways to fulfil their needs and compare them to how they fulfilled these when offending. It allows the offender to have a basic grasp of what has caused their sexually abusive behaviour. On the one hand, it is important to help them understand what has led them to their offending, but on the other hand, it is imperative that they feel safe enough to explore their past deviant behaviour. This encourages them to feel at ease, free from judgment and condemnation. For the one hour while in therapeutic engagement, the therapist should help them break down the barriers to their sense of self. Accepting responsibility for their actions comes later, always, but at the beginning, it is offering them a sense of safety.

Grief work

Much of the earlier therapeutic work is exploring loss. There will be men who are estranged from their families often moving back to their parents. Some are suicidal and it's not uncommon for them to seek out ways to do this. I had one client who bought everything he needed online to end his life humanely with little discomfort, although he didn't go on to do it. In general, suicidal urges do seem to fade over time.

Jack's story Part 2: Session 23

It is five months since the day of the knock. Jack feels better but is still apprehensive about what the future holds for him. He and his wife Jenny are getting on better, and Jenny has decided to stand by Jack until the case is concluded. She feels there is hope for the marriage and has allowed him to return home. Although she is still struggling with her issues of trust, overall, their relationship is better. Jack has not heard anything from the police or his solicitor. One of the difficult challenges for our clients is the waiting. They often feel in limbo, unable to move on until it's over. Jack has been extremely committed to therapy, even though he has found it difficult to talk about his past.

Over 23 sessions, Jack has explored his childhood timeline and journey of addiction to pornography. In the seventh therapy session, Jack informed David that he was abused by his father's friend Ted, who was a farmer. From the age of seven, Jack would go to collect newly laid eggs from Ted's farm. Ted was married but his wife never seemed to be there when he visited. He later found out that the farmer would always make sure that his wife was out when Jack visited. Not long after he started visiting him, he fell over and scuffed his knee. It was bleeding and Ted said, 'Come here and I will make it better for you'. Ted took him upstairs and laid him on the bed. He washed his hands in the sink in the bedroom before sitting next to him. Ted then started licking his cut knee and Jack told him that it felt strange what he was doing but it felt nice at the same time, apart from that horrible smell. When David asked what the smell was, Jack said Ted had terrible body odour. Jack had said that this was the start of the sexual abuse. Jack had admitted in an earlier session that he once thought that he was in love with Ted. Apart from abusing Jack, they would play games together, something his father never did. He could talk to Ted about how he was feeling, and Ted would always be kind and tell him that he could tell him anything.

One day when Jack was 14, he and Ted argued, and Jack stormed out of the farm informing him that he would not be seeing him again. He had started to wonder if he was gay, but was confused because he was also attracted to a girl at school. He noticed that over the past few months, he had started to become irritated with Ted and was aware he wasn't being very kind to him. Jack eventually realised that what Ted was doing was wrong and that he was sexually abusing him. He once asked Ted if he had been abused as a child. Ted scorned him and told him that he wasn't abusing him and that it was a mutual love they had for each other. A few days after the argument, he informed his parents of Ted abusing him and his father got angry saying that he was lying and sent him to his room. Ted and his father had been good friends for many years, and Jack was aware that Ted had helped his father out financially when he was out of work.

Jack was now 34 and Ted was now in his seventies. Twelve months ago, it became known that two other men had reported Ted to the police for historical sexual abuse. Because of his current situation, Jack was uncertain of reporting him as he felt that if his conviction were to be in the newspaper it might cause other issues. In the previous session, Jack had explored reporting Ted to the police.

At the beginning of each session, David checks in with Jack.

David: Jack, I was wondering if there was anything left over from our session last week that you wanted to explore.

Jack: I found last week's session to be difficult, talking about Ted again. Then this week while I was at work, I was offloading a delivery and when the driver gave me the delivery note.

> I nearly heaved as he stank of BO, I grabbed the delivery note off him and walked off. I couldn't stop thinking of Ted; he smelt of him.
>
> David: That one moment had you laired by Ted again, is it that's how it felt?
>
> Jack: Yes, all day I was consumed by him, errrhhh! *Jack grimaced with disgust.*
>
> David: That smell took you back to him, almost back to the scene of the crime, is that what happened to you?
>
> Jack: Yes.
>
> *Jack went quiet.*

What is the rationale for abusive behaviour? There may be a variety of reasons why an individual would commit this sort of offence. However, there are some common denominators that I will touch upon and will also be explored in other chapters.

Sexual addiction

Addictive behaviour is when an individual is struggling with a compulsion and is unable to stop the compulsion. For years people have thought that an addiction is when someone struggles with issues around drugs, alcohol, and gambling, but since the introduction of the internet, more addictive behaviours have emerged, such as gaming (Liu et al., 2017) and pornography. Addiction can be defined as an individual who is struggling to cease a particular behaviour whether desiring to or not. Sexual addiction is often referred to in different terms, such as Hypersexual Disorder (HD), Compulsive Sexual Behaviour (CSB), and Compulsive Sexual Behaviour Disorder (CSBD) which has now been included in ICD-11 as an impulse control disorder. That said, there is still an ongoing debate on whether sex addiction is a real thing (Pistre et al., 2023). Carnes et al. (2014) argued that sexual addiction is a valid concept, while Swan (2016) and Neves (2021) argued that sex addiction doesn't exist. Kerner (2014) suggested that at present, there is a lack of evidence-based research on the subject to prove that it is an addiction. Attention Deficit Hyperactivity Disorder (ADHD) can also play a part in sexual addiction. In a recent review, Sahithya and Kashyap suggested that 'Sexual addiction disorder often presents with comorbid disorders such as anxiety, mood disorders, substance abuse and ADHD' (Sahithya & Kashyap, 2022, p. 96).

Pornography addiction

Pornography addiction is a relatively new terminology that is used to describe someone who views pornography excessively. Before the explosion of the world wide web in 1994, it would be difficult to define someone as having a pornography addiction because of the difficulty in obtaining such content. In those days, pornography was illegal in the UK, with only 'soft pornography' available to purchase from sex shops.

The dopamine factor

When considering addiction, one must look at various regions of the brain that contribute to it: the frontal and dorsolateral cortex being the most sophisticated areas, responsible for decision-making. The Basal forebrain section controls the area of the body's reward system and controls survival instincts. The Ventral Tegmental Area (VTA) of the midbrain is where the chemical messenger dopamine is produced. Dopamine is a neurotransmitter, or a neuromodulator, a chemical messenger that plays a role in various functions, including motivation, feelings of pleasure and motor control. It also plays a critical role in addiction. If individuals do something that they consider rewarding, such as eating food, smoking a cigarette, or having sex, dopamine neurons are released into the VTA and activated, making the person want to do it again.

There has been much research (Hall, 2013) on the chemical messenger systems such as dopamine and noradrenaline with evidence that they are necessary to the mechanism of addiction. Hall stated that 'pleasure is not purely psychological, but a physical process triggered by chemicals in the brain. . . . dopamine, endorphins and adrenaline' (Hall, 2013, p. 12). Sexual activity creates a feeling of pleasure, which feeds the striatum and energises motivation. Gary Wilson (2014) argued that pornography is an addiction similar to overeating and gambling.

If an individual has high levels of sexual activity, it will cause dopamine to surge repeatedly towards the decision-making area of the brain. One notable reason for this is a continuing increase of the protein ΔFosB, which is more commonly known as DeltaFosB. DeltaFosB is a transcription factor that plays a pivotal role in regulating natural behaviours such as a response to food or sex, and is a splice variant that triggers the development of addiction. It acts as a molecular switch that enhances the sensitivity of neurons to dopamine. The more someone watches pornography, the more DeltaFosB accumulates, because of its unusual protein stabilities (Nestler, 2014).

DeltaFosB is a highly stable protein that, once overexpressed by recurrent choice behaviours, leads to an addictive state (Nestler, 2001). The brain has millions of neural pathways and some of these pathways are specifically responsible for feelings of pleasure. If these pathways are overexposed to pleasure, the stronger the connection becomes. Neural pathways are where habits are formed and the stronger the pathway becomes, the more it becomes 'less effective' (Hall, 2013) so losing their 'desired effect'. When this happens, the addict requires more stimulation, creating an addiction cycle.

Overconsumption results in the molecular switch being activated (Nestler, 2012) and once activated, new gene expressions become influential and changes in synapses occur. It is thought that the build-up of the DeltaFosB protein remains present for one to two months after the impulsive behaviour has ceased by the addict (Nestler, 2012), continuing to stimulate compulsive behaviour and impacting sensitisation. The client needs to understand that the more they watch pornography, the more they will crave dopamine (Starcke et al., 2018). From a pornography addiction perspective, this can sometimes lead to the person watching it for many hours a day, seeking and searching for that next video or image and over time becoming more desensitised.

A comparison may therefore be made between what happens in the brain when an individual consumes an excessive quantity of fatty and/or sugary foods with what happens when they engage in high levels of sexual activity. In both cases, levels of dopamine become chronically high and this causes DeltaFosB (Nestler, 2001) to build up in the brain. As the addiction develops, more of a dopamine hit is needed to increase the sexual stimuli to affect the sexual response, therefore, the male viewer can develop pornography-induced erectile dysfunction (PIED) (Kirby, 2021). As the craving for something more exciting develops, the more difficult it is to maintain an erection, thus making it difficult to achieve orgasm or experience pleasurable sensations during sexual activity with a partner.

Death-grip syndrome

Death-grip syndrome is a term used to describe a phenomenon where men experience a decrease in sensitivity during sexual activity due to overstimulation from masturbation with a tight grip or excessive pressure. The high intensity of pressure needed to reach 'nirvana' can often be difficult to replicate during penetrative sex. Not recognised as an official medical condition, the term 'death-grip syndrome' implies that the tight grip or pressure used during masturbation can 'kill' or decrease sensitivity in the penis, leading to difficulties in sexual function and satisfaction. When individuals masturbate with a tight grip or apply excessive pressure, they may experience heightened sensations and achieve orgasm more quickly. The grip of a hand will be firmer than that of a vagina or anus and this can create a distorted perception of what is considered normal or desirable in real-life sexual experiences and can have an impact on sexual satisfaction within a relationship and overall well-being. When someone becomes accustomed to the intense stimulation provided by pornography, they may find it challenging to derive satisfaction from real-life sexual experiences with their partners. This can result in feelings of dissatisfaction, frustration, and even resentment within the relationship. Moreover, the emphasis on physical gratification in pornography can overshadow the emotional and relational aspects of intimacy. This can lead individuals to prioritise physical pleasure over emotional connection and intimacy within their relationships. As he becomes more dissatisfied, the feelings of inadequacy or insecurity for both partners can start to create a sexual disconnect.

It is not uncommon for addicts to try to manipulate their partner into acting out their sexual fantasies that have been created from the viewing of pornography.

Initially, their partner may play out their fantasies but over time will become dissatisfied with the sexual relationship and question its boundaries. This dynamic can lead to conflicts and challenges within a relationship, often resulting in one partner feeling pressured or manipulated to fulfil the desires of the other. This can create feelings of emotional intimacy being lost, resentful, hurt, and betrayed.

Besides its impact on partners, these same neurological principles apply when addiction itself originates in trauma, or where attachment disruptions have similar neurological effects (Hudson-Allez, 2011). For example, shame is a common obstacle in clients understanding their addictions. Gilliland emphasised the importance of understanding shame's origins, stating that 'hypersexual behaviour may be engaged as a maladaptive substitute or deflection of existing shame rather than seeing shame only as the result of such behaviour' (Gilliland, et al., 2011, p. 6).

So why do some people become more addicted to pornography than others? One could ask the same question about drugs, alcohol, or gambling. In general, it can be a variety of things, such as unresolved mental health issues, anxiety, or depression. Over time the addict will move to other ways to satisfy their sexual urges and it is often by chance that they end up engaging in online secret behaviour. They may seek out escorts, or hook-ups online, and quite often use online internet platforms to engage in sexual conversation, commonly with other men. Without realising it, the addict is then stepping into a danger zone of crossing the line.

As with other addictions, the sexual behaviours of individuals suffering from sex or pornography addiction can be defined as coping mechanisms or escapism (Becker, Perry, & Westenbroek, 2012) to free the person from the emotional pain of life or past traumatic experiences. Such escapism, however, contradicts its objective as it creates a cycle of increasing desperation, shame, and preoccupation. Hall suggests that there is no 'single or simple answer' (Hall, 2013, p. 33) that determines why an individual develops an addiction. In my experience, if a client can start to understand their addiction and how it originated, they may be able to reflect more positively about their past and avoid other possible addictive behaviours allowing them to discuss more openly while in therapy.

The drama triangle

The more an individual acts out sexually the more they will disregard any of the possible consequences that may happen to them. A person suffering from addiction will undoubtedly have formed cognitive distortions about themselves, which are not helpful or productive. This is partly illustrated by Karpman (2007) in his 'drama triangle' model. The drama triangle is a concept that describes dysfunctional interactions among people. It involves three roles: the victim, the rescuer, and the persecutor. The rescuer tries to save or fix the victim, who then feels oppressed or powerless, so persecutes, blames or criticises the rescuer. The roles can be fluid with the individual switching between all of them, perpetuating the drama.

So, what does this look like in an addict?

- *Victim role*: the addict may perceive themselves as a victim of circumstance, genetics, or past traumas, feeling powerless to their addiction and unable to help themselves without support from others.
- *Rescuer role*: family or friends may take the role of the rescuers by enabling the addictive behaviour, attempting to shield the addict from the consequences, or trying to fix the problem.
- *Persecutor role*: other people in the addict's life, including family and friends, may adopt a persecutor role, by blaming, shaming, and criticising them, thus reinforcing their feelings of guilt and shame.

These roles can create dysfunctional thinking leading to cognitive dissonance because of contrasting beliefs. Shame can also play a major role in an addict's behaviour and act as a driver of the addiction.

One approach to the work is Internalized-Other-Interviewing (IOI), a practice promoted by Tomm (2017) which has its origins in family therapy. This approach links with concepts found in psychoanalysis and could be useful in therapy. It can be valuable when attempting to assist a client suffering from sexual addiction to understand how their condition impacts their partner. Drawing on the work of the psychoanalyst Freud (1920), it is important to examine the causes and consequences of sexual addiction and suggest other approaches that could re-establish their relationships. It's important to address any previous traumas that may have played a part in their behaviour, this will help them look at themselves more positively and recognise defects in their cognitive thinking.

It is common for psychological distress to continue while in recovery which can lead to relapse, (Hasin et al., 2002) nonetheless, the client will have learned sufficient tools (Hall, 2013) to support their journey of beating sex addiction. Other psychological motivations may contribute to their behaviour such as curiosity, arousal, or seeking novelty.

As I mentioned earlier, becoming desensitised to pornography leads to seeking something more sexually satisfying. Additionally, societal influences such as cultural attitudes towards sex and masculinity, as well as accessibility and anonymity afforded by the internet, may play a role. Furthermore, some individuals may have underlying issues such as cross-addictions that drive their behaviour, as already discussed. It's crucial to recognise that each case is unique, and understanding the multifaceted nature of this behaviour requires more research.

Repetition compulsion

Another reason that an individual commits this sort of offence is repetition compulsion (Hudson-Allez, 2011). This is a concept where individuals unconsciously repeat patterns of behaviour or experiences which are reminiscent of past traumatic events in childhood. This unconscious trait was first introduced by Freud (1914).

He suggested that it can derive from physical, emotional, and sexual abuse. An example would be an individual unconsciously seeking out toxic relationships repeatedly. Patrick Carnes suggested that early sexual experiences shape our perception of what arouses and attracts us, forming a 'storyline' that influences our preferences. From these encounters, a narrative develops, intertwining elements that we associate with sexual arousal (Carnes, 2018).

Jack's story Part 3: Session 67

Jack has been to magistrates' court and his case has been pushed up to crown court. This is not uncommon as solicitors seem to favour this happening, simply because the judges in crown court are more familiar with these offences.

David: Jack, your case is finally coming to an end, so it will soon be over. I have to say, you seemed quite calm on our last session the day before the Magistrates' court.

Jack: Yes, I was nervous of course but that is to be expected. As I told you, my solicitor thinks that at worst it will be a suspended sentence, but we are hoping for a community order. If it's a suspended sentence, well, I can live with that. After all, I did do it, so I have to accept what comes my way. Fingers crossed that that's the worst it's going to be.

David: I think that you have done really well on this journey, and you seem to be much happier in who you are as a person, which seems very different to the Jack I first met.

Jack: Yes, it's strange, isn't it? I think that I have changed a lot and I don't sweat over the small stuff anymore.

David: Why do you feel that you can cope better?

Jack: I think facing my anger towards Ted. I never realised how much he still had a hold over me. I am pleased that I never reported him. That would have just dragged it on; the other accusations should be enough to send him down. I am at peace with it now. Jack paused and then went on, although I take full responsibility, I can't help thinking that if I hadn't been abused and he never introduced me to porn at such a young age, I wouldn't have had to go through this and I wouldn't have had that thing you mentioned, what was it – something compulsion?

David: Repetition compulsion?

> Jack: Yes, that's it.
>
> *In this session, Jack shows his elements of reflection and accept-*
> *ance. He has accepted that his offending was directly linked to*
> *the childhood abuse from Ted and his introduction to pornography*
> *at the age of just nine years old.*

Persistence rather than desistance

Why do individuals persist in engaging in illegal behaviour online? When discussing this issue with clients, I often pose a hypothetical scenario: if offered a free week-long trip to New York City, with the caveat that the city has been devoid of law enforcement for over a decade, rampant with violence orchestrated by various gangs, including daily occurrences of murder, rape, and widespread looting, and streets deserted, would they still choose to visit? The unanimous response is of course no. Consequently, it begs the question: why then, do individuals knowingly jeopardize their own lives, future, family, friendships, and livelihoods by engaging in illicit activities online?

Dissecting why an individual views child sexual abuse material (CSAM) online can be complex and long-winded. It needs the therapist to be patient and persistent in the phenomenological enquiries. It is while delving into their timeline, unravelling their story, and addressing the client's past right up to the day of the knock. Exploring any possible root causes will allow the client to navigate their way through the complex maze on route to their understanding. We often use a trauma-informed approach and help them achieve this. Cognitive Behavioural Therapy (CBT) tools are also used along with various handouts each week for homework. We play a vital role in their rehabilitation and desistance. The long-term hope is for our client to cease engaging in any future online illegal behaviour and help navigate their own change and move forward to more a positive and fulfilling life on their journey to transformation and autonomy.

Our work extends beyond our therapy sessions. A therapist will need to incorporate a much broader understanding of what their client is facing, such as the court process, social services, court orders and the criminal justice system terminology. You will be collaborating with legal professionals, psychologists, and sometimes other family members.

The general public's view

The perception of psychotherapists who work with people who commit sexual offences in the UK varies among the general public. Some may view these professionals with scepticism or even disdain, associating them closely with the individuals they treat and perhaps questioning the ethics of providing therapy to those who have committed such serious offences. This has happened to me on numerous occasions, so I now choose not to tell people what I do. I once asked a colleague about his stance on this issue, and he said that he tells them that he works in a supermarket stacking shelves. It's not all bad though, as there is also recognition among many that therapy for people who commit sexual offences can play a crucial role in rehabilitation and reducing the risk of reoffending. Those who understand the importance of rehabilitation may view these psychotherapists as valuable contributors to public safety and rehabilitation efforts. Overall, perceptions may depend on individuals' understanding of the complexities of sexual offending, their attitudes towards rehabilitation and punishment, and their trust in the effectiveness of psychotherapy in addressing such challenging issues.

Conclusion

In summary, I have explored the journey of an individual who crosses the boundary into viewing CSAM on the internet. I have discussed the implications of the 'knock' and its consequences, examining various factors that may lead someone down this path. These include sexual addiction, pornography addiction driven by dopamine, and repetition compulsion from early childhood trauma. Additionally, I have addressed the issues of sexual dysfunction and relationship difficulties faced by those who excessively consume online pornography. Through a case study, I have provided an insight into the challenges a counsellor and/or therapist may face when working with this client group plus illustrating how they might approach this challenging work.

References

Becker, J., Perry A., & Westenbroek C. (2012) Sex differences in the neural mechanisms mediating addiction: a new synthesis and hypothesis. https://bsd.biomedcentral.com/articles/10.1186/2042-6410-3-14.

Carnes, P. J. (2018) *Out of the Shadows: Understanding Sexual Addictions.* Hazelden Trade.

Carnes, P. J., Hopkins, T. A., & Green, B. A. (2014) Clinical relevance of the proposed sexual addiction diagnostic criteria: relation to Sexual Addiction Screening Test-revised. *Journal of Addictive Medicine* 8(6), 450–461. doi:10.1097/ADM.0000000000000080. PMID:25303984.

Erskine, R., Moursund, J. P., & Trautmann, R. L. (2023) *Beyond Empathy.* Routledge.

Freud, S. (1914) Remembering, repeating and working through. In *The standard edition of the complete psychological works of Sigmund Freud, Vol XII* (1911–1913): *The case of Schreber, papers on technique & other works* (pp. 145–156). Hogarth Press.

Freud, S. (1920) *Beyond the Pleasure Principle* (Standard Edition, Vol. 18, pp. 7–64). Hogarth.

Gilliland, R., South, M., Carpenter, B. N., & Hardy, S. A., (2011). The roles of shame and guilt in hypersexual behaviour. *Sexual Addiction & Compulsivity, 18*(1), 6.

Hall, P. (2013) *Understanding and treating sex and pornography addiction.* Routledge.

Hasin, D., Liu, X. & Nunes, E., McCloud, S. Sarnet, S., & Endicott, J. (2002) Effects of major depression on remission and relapse of substance dependence. *Archives of General Psychiatry, 59*(4), 375–380. doi:10.1001/archpsyc.59.4.375.

Hudson-Allez, G. (2011) *Infant losses, adult searches: A neural and developmental perspective on psychotherapy and sexual offending.* 2nd ed. Routledge.

ICD11 (2022) International Statistical Classification of Diseases and Related Health Problems. www.who.int/standards/classifications/classification-of-diseases

Karpman, S. (2007) The new drama triangles. https://karpmandramatriangle.com/pdf/thenew dramatriangles.pdf.

Kerner, I. (2014) Is sex addiction real? Depends on whom you ask. https://edition.cnn. com/2016/12/14/health/sex-addiction-real-or-not-kerner/index.html.

Kirby, M. (2021) Pornography and its impact on the sexual health of men. *Trends Urology & Men Health,* 12, 6–10. https://doi.org/10.1002/tre.791

Liu, L., Yip, S. W., Zhang, J.-T., Wang, L-J., Shen, Z. J., & Liu, B. (2017) Activation of the ventral and dorsal stratum during cue reactivity in Internet gaming disorder. *Addiction Biology*, 22(3), 791–801. Doi:10.1111/adb.12338.

Neves, S. (2021) *Compulsive Sexual Behaviours: A Psycho-Sexual Treatment Guide for Clinicians*. Routledge.

Nestler, E. J. (2001) Molecular basis of long-term plasticity underlying addiction. *Nature Reviews Neuroscience* 2(2), 119–128 doi:10.1038/35053570.

Nestler, E. J. (2012) Transcriptional mechanisms of drug addiction. *Clinical Psychopharmocology and Neuroscience,* 10(3), 136–143. doi:10.9758/cpn.2012.10.3.136

Nestler, E. J. (2014) Epigenic mechanisms of drug addiction. *Neuropharmacology,* 76, Pt B, 259–268. DOI:10.1016/j.neuropharm.2013.04.004.

Pistre, N., Schreck, B., Gall-Bronnec, M., & Fatseas, M. (2023) Should problematic sexual behaviour be viewed under the scope of addiction? A systematic review based on DSM-5 substance use disorder criteria. *Addictive Behaviors Reports*, 18, 100510. https://doi. org/10.1016/j.abrep.2023.100510.

Sahithya, B. R. & Kashyap, R. S. (2022) Sexual addiction disorder – A review with recent updates. *Journal of Psychosexual Health*, 4(2), 95–101.

Starcke, K., Antons, S., Trotke, P., & Brand, M., (2018). Cue-reactivity in behavioural addictions: A meta-analysis and methodological considerations. *Journal of Behavioural Addictions*, 7(2), 227–238.

Swan, J. (2016) Anthony Weiner Is Not a Sex Addict, Neither Is Anyone Else. https:// www.psychologytoday.com/gb/blog/close-and-personal/201609/anthony-weiner-is-not-sex-addict-neither-is-anyone-else-0.

Tomm, K. (2017) Internalised-Other-Interviewing. www.commonlamguagepsychotherapy. org. https://www.commonlanguagepsychotherapy.org/assets/accepted_procedures/inter nalizedotherinterv.pdf.

Ward, T., Hudson, S. M., & Keenan, T. (1998). A self-regulation model of the sexual offense process, *Sexual Abuse: Journal of Research and Treatment*, 10(2), 141–157. https://doi. org/10.1023/A:1022071516644.

Ward, T. & Stewart, C. A. (2003) Good lives and the rehabilitation of sexual offenders. In T. Ward, R. Laws, & S. M. Hudson (eds) *Sexual Deviance: Issues and Controversies* (pp. 21–44). Sage.

Wilson, G. (2014) *Your Brain on Porn*. Commonwealth.

Chapter 8

'Do I stay or do I go?!'
The non-offending partner

Trudy Hannington

Introduction

Undertaking therapeutic work with a non-offending partner (NOP) of a person who has committed a sexual offence is hugely complex. I hear so many people say, 'if my partner did that, I would definitely leave'. However, the reality isn't quite the same. Staying with a partner often promotes judgement and alienation from outsiders, not just from the general public, but also from those closest to them, such as their dearest friends and their closest family. This alienates NOPs further and, in some ways, makes it even more difficult to leave as they would then have no support network. NOPs often avoid making new friends for fear of them finding out, or being judged, or having to tell others what has happened if they have children, because of the restrictions and declarations that are imposed as part of sentencing. The ripple effect is huge, with the partner suffering a sentence just as much as the offender.

Whilst there is limited research about the non-offending partner, what there is clearly evidences that they suffer significant repercussions following the discovery of their partner's crimes. After the knock, they suffer grief, trauma and social isolation. However, the NOPs support needs have typically been overlooked, with priority instead placed on equipping NOPs with the skills to monitor their partner's behaviour and/or protect their children from sexual abuse (Duncan et al., 2020).

This chapter will give an overview of working with the NOP, whether they choose to stay or to leave. I will explore the different areas of concern and potential implication for themselves, their children, their wider family, and their friends. I will also discuss the social stigma associated with this type of crime and the potential changes to the NOPs' future lives.

I finish with a discussion of the importance of self-care for the therapist when working with the NOP.

Working with the partner who chooses to stay

As therapists, we strive to be non-judgemental and empathic, but when working with the non-offending partner, we hear the stories of what their partners have done and it can then be difficult to understand why a NOP would want to stay with a

DOI: 10.4324/9781003509103-10

sex offender. The majority of referrals to StopSO, and what is a growing concern nationally with approximately 850 arrests per month, is the escalation of regular pornography use moving to downloading child sexual abuse material (CSAM) (Centre of Expertise, 2023).

Some may have escalated into watching videos of the sexual abuse of children or talking to them in chat rooms, and grooming them to meet for sex. Seen less often at StopSO, but may also happen, are offences that include the sharing of naked images of their own children, or their friends' children, in order to get the same from other offenders in return. On other occasions it might be that the husband or partner has perhaps been sexual with their own child or children.

As a therapist, when you hear the words from a NOP, 'I love him, I can't leave him', it can be very difficult to comprehend, no matter how non-judgemental we strive to be. Therefore, good supervision is vital if you are considering this type of work. Offering therapy to a partner who chooses to stay with someone who has committed a sexual offence is a very delicate and complex process. It requires listening with empathy even when the person is getting into the details of the offence; this is often a really important part of the process as you are likely to be the only person in their lives that they can tell the truth to.

Creating a safe space and warm environment for the NOP to share their story, validating their feelings through active listening, acknowledging without judgement or interruption their reasons for staying, hearing their fears and doubts about the potential future, all play a huge part in their healing process. It is also important that you don't minimise or try to help them make excuses for what has happened. No matter what else is going on in his life, there will never be a valid reason for abusing children, and as therapists, we need to keep this foremost in our minds. We also need to communicate this, once again without judgement, as it is important that we do not collude with what has happened.

'Rita'

Rita's partner John was arrested for chatting online to a girl aged 13 and arranging to meet her for 'kissing and fish and chips at the seaside'. Rita said, 'he only did it because he was lonely. I was being treated for breast cancer and I was just so tired all the time and we weren't having sex anymore!'. John's argument was 'I didn't mean any harm. I'm young at heart, like Peter Pan!' The 13-year-old girl turned out to be an undercover 'sting' by the police. When Rita related the story in therapy she said, 'there wasn't even a child involved, it was a police officer not a real child'. In my experience, the non-offending partner will also minimise, make excuses or even blame themselves in order to accept and live with what he has done.

It is vital that a clear confidentiality agreement is established prior to starting the therapy with a NOP and that this is discussed and understood by the client. I always find the following quote from Dr Andrew Smith extremely helpful to keep in mind:

> I am aware as a therapist/counsellor of my primary responsibility for maintaining confidentiality between myself and the client. However, this general rule of confidentiality can be broken if you disclose information about a criminal offence or conduct that puts others or yourself at serious risk of harm. An attempt would be made to talk to you before disclosure if this does not further compromise anybody's personal safety.
>
> (Smith, 2022, p. 6)

Given that in 2021, there were over 850 arrests a month across the UK for accessing child sexual abuse material, many of these individuals would have had children of their own or in their wider family. Compared to other types of sexual offending, people who access child sexual abuse material are more likely to be married and have children (Centre of Expertise, 2023).

Smith also goes on to suggest that counselling partners of offenders can be divided into three categories:

1. Counselling partners where there are no safeguarding risk management issues.
2. Counselling partners in order to improve their safeguarding ability to protect children from sexual abuse.
3. Counselling partners and other family members in a systematic way to consolidate and enhance family safety.

This will help you to keep an awareness of safeguarding and confidentiality at each session as standard practice.

Despite the betrayal and the trauma the knock has caused, the NOP does not just fall out of love with their partner overnight. Religious beliefs around marriage may play a part, believing that they have to stay, as they promised marriage for life. The NOP may have strong emotional ties to their partner, making it difficult to leave no matter how severe the offence. They may feel torn by what their partner has done versus the love they feel and the attachment they have to their partner.

If we explore this from a trauma-bonding perspective, in the context of a non-offending partner staying with a partner who has committed a sexual offence, it can help us to understand what else might be happening. Trauma-bonding refers to the strong emotional connection that can develop between individuals who have experienced traumatic events together, even if one person has caused harm to the other. In this scenario, the non-offending partner may have endured various forms of manipulation, coercion, or abuse from the offender, leading to a complex blend of emotions including fear, love, and loyalty. Despite the harmful actions of the offender, the NOP may feel deeply attached and connected due to shared experiences of trauma and survival. This bond can create a powerful psychological pull, making it exceedingly difficult for the NOP to leave the relationship, for fear of losing the emotional connection, or struggling with feelings of guilt and responsibility (Salter, Woodlock, & Jones, 2023). Understanding trauma-bonding is essential for therapists working with non-offending partners, as it helps us to understand the complexity of their experiences and can help inform appropriate therapeutic interventions.

'Angela'

Angela stayed with her partner, choosing to believe him over her child, who said daddy was touching her. The child was four years old and was taken into care and subsequently adopted. The child chose to find her mum at the age of 24 to ask why she didn't believe her. The wider story was that Angela was in a domestic violent situation and the manipulation and coercion from her husband meant that she stayed with him. She did not recall any questions being asked or investigations being made about her situation; she was judged alongside the offender. She said she didn't feel she had a voice. Angela came from a very dysfunctional family and remembered her own mother would encourage the husband to beat her up if she ever dared answer him back, arguing the little girl had made it up to escape from her.

Victim blaming

Often the offender will promise to do anything to make things better, offering to go to therapy, making excuses for their behaviour or denying it completely; maybe even blaming their partner for why they have done what they've done. This can all add to the confusion of such a big decision to make as to whether to stay or whether to leave. It is important as a therapist that you are mindful of potential coercion toward the NOP by the offender as this can be quite subtle. Sometimes, the NOP can change their mind about staying on a week-by-week, day-by-day, hour-by-hour, and minute-by-minute basis, so it can be quite hard to keep up. Once again, the therapist needs to be mindful of the importance of staying where the client is at, in their process, as well as what is happening in the here-and-now, which might be influencing it too.

It is widely documented that those arrested and/or charged with a sexual offence are at increased risk of suicide and this is often emphasised to the NOP by the offender. This can put a lot of guilt and pressure on the NOP to stay with the partner, the NOP believing their partner can't possibly survive without them. Sometimes the offender's family puts pressure on the NOP to stay as they fear that the offender will commit suicide if they lose their partner and their children

(Steel et al., 2022). There is also further evidence that demonstrates that recidivism rates are lower for those who are in a healthy, romantic relationship, once again potentially adding more pressure on the NOP to stay (Lytle, Bailey, & Bensel, 2017).

Financial worries can also put partners under a lot of pressure to stay. If a NOP is financially dependent on their partner and has no other support network, it can feel impossible to leave or to ask their partner to leave. It might be that the offender has lost their job, so they are financially dependent on the NOP. It is also extremely difficult for the NOP to leave their lovely home, or take their children away from their home. Most NOPs do not want to tell their children what their father (in most cases) has done, because of the impact on them (Stop It Now, 2024).

Children are a huge concern if the NOP chooses to stay. Sometimes social services will remove the children (see Chapter 4), even if they weren't the victims of the crime that has been committed. This can be even more isolating and discriminating for the NOP, being blamed for the children being removed. It is common for the authorities to expect that the NOP will have the responsibility of keeping the children safe, monitoring the offender partner's behaviour, and monitoring their internet use if the charges are for online offences. The offender may not be able to take their children to school, or ever see them in a school production again. They may not be able to take them to the park, take them swimming, or any other activities where other children might be. Even places to go for holidays will also be restricted.

Guilt by association

In some cases, if the NOP works with children or vulnerable adults they have to inform their employer of their partner's sexual offences, and in some cases the NOP may lose their own jobs because they have chosen to stay with the offender. Although the NOP and their children have not committed an offence, they are punished by the system nevertheless.

It is also well documented that NOPs often suffer with PTSD, anxiety, and depression as a result of not only the shock of what their partner has done, but the repercussions that then unfold as time goes on. Sadly, it never goes away whether they stay or whether they go (Cahalane & Duff, 2017).

Pressure from friends and family to leave the offender is most common. There might be total disbelief that they would even consider staying with a sex offender. Family and friends often distance themselves for fear of their own reputation: 'guilt by association'. There might be other children with friends and the wider family, which then adds further restrictions and more potential investigations, so it can be the offender and the NOP that choose to alienate themselves from family and friends (Lytle, Bailey, & Bensel, 2017). This a real concern for the NOP as this just isolates them even further.

The local community may find out what has happened, possibly because vigilantes are involved, or the heavy police early morning visit from 'the knock' gets the curtains twitching. It may be reported in the press, which usually happens when the offender is someone who is seen as a pillar of the community. This is then usually shared on social media so the news can reach far and wide. The repercussions for the NOP and the children can be profound; they often face judgement and are stigmatised by the community, associating them with the crime of the offender. This just exacerbates the shame, guilt, and fear for the NOP and the children. This can make it difficult to reach out for help and support even from professionals. There may also be difficulties on a practical level, finding alternative accommodation, financial support, and legal implications, particularly in cases involving child access and/or child protection services, which are just the start of the hurdles to be faced.

Loss of technology

When 'the knock' happens, the police often confiscate all technology. This not only means taking the alleged offenders' electronic devices, but may also mean they take the kids and the NOPs electronic devices which can include phones, PCs, laptops, iPads, cameras, and games consoles. Some are never returned, so this can mean the loss of family photos that can never be replaced, personal information being seen, or even impact on the NOP's work or the children's homework, despite being innocent victims.

Client referrals

At the moment there is limited help available for the NOP, the children, and the wider family that is free to access. Most support is either authority involvement or privately paid for therapeutic interventions. Therefore, it is vitally important for you to actively encourage an NOP to develop their own self-care package. I had a client only recently who ended up being sectioned under the mental health act as a result of the outcome of her partner's court case; she was totally unprepared for the possible outcome at court. She had not sought or been offered any help whilst they had waited over two years for the case to be heard. They had lived what appeared to be a very 'normal' life with no interference from authorities, so it was a huge shock when the offender was told that they would now be on the sex offender's register for ten years and how this would impact both of their lives. Most other crimes receive a punishment that is either completed by a prison sentence, or court orders, with little or no involvement from anyone after sentencing. However, with sex offences registration goes on for years after the sentencing, being checked up on and being judged, making it difficult for the couple to put it behind them and move on.

As a therapist you may see the non-offending partner at any part of the criminal justice journey. It may be straight after 'the knock' when their house has been raided by the police at 5am. Or it may be when social services swoop in and threaten to take their children away if the NOP stays with the offender. Often, as months go by, they are in limbo as to when the next step of the criminal justice process will occur. Sometimes, post-sentencing is when reality for the NOP really hits, given that the average time for these types of cases to be brought to court is two, possibly three years. In that time, the NOP can lull themselves into a false sense of security that it's all been forgotten, so when the court case does happen, the reality really does overwhelm them as everything seems to happen very quickly from this time. Probation visits, police visits, social services visits, can sometimes be daily depending on the case.

Sexual relationship

A convicted partner can have a huge impact on the intimacy of the couple. The NOP may feel they have to be really sexual all of the time, in order to prevent the offender 'acting out' and offending again. This can be reinforced with questioning on post-conviction police visits. I had a client recently who chose to stay with their partner and post-sentence, the police asked them if they were having sex, how often they were being sexual, and what type of sex they were having. She felt judged by the police officers and it made her question whether they were thinking that what her partner had done must somehow be her fault, for not giving him enough sex or good enough sex. Many women question themselves in this same way; was it their fault their partners had looked at CSAM, because they weren't having enough sex or the type of sex their partner wanted or needed? They question 'is it because I'm getting older and he really wants sex with someone younger?'. This can have a huge impact on the NOP's self-esteem and sexuality.

There is often a high level of sexual dysfunction in this situation and this can be for both the NOP and the offender. The therapist can help the NOP explore their concerns, fears, and anxieties around resuming sexual activity. It is also useful to explore their boundaries and for the NOP to relay those boundaries to her partner in order to help facilitate the rebuilding of trust and help prevent triggers and setbacks. Some NOPs say they get intrusive thoughts and images of what their partners have done when they attempt to be intimate again. A therapist can help the NOP to develop coping strategies to manage flashbacks, triggers, and other distressing symptoms that can arise when attempting to be intimate again (Duncan, et al., 2022). Being sexual again with an offending partner is probably one of the most difficult areas I cover with a client, as they often feel guilty for even wanting to be sexual again and it may be beneficial to encourage clients to attend couple therapy with a trained psychosexual therapist involved in forensic work (StopSO. org.uk; COSRT.org.uk).

Couple therapy

Depending on the circumstances, the therapist may also work with the couple to address the offender's behaviour, encouraging them to take responsibility for their actions, and participate in treatment programmes aimed at reducing the risk of reoffending. Couple therapy can be extremely helpful once the NOP feels ready, and this can help the couple to start over, attempting to draw a line and leave what has happened in the past in order to move on to a more positive future. This can also help them rebuild trust, establish boundaries, improve communication, and develop healthier patterns of relating to each other.

Discovering that their partner is a sex offender can severely damage trust within the relationship. A therapist can help an NOP explore what they need to rebuild their trust, by giving a safe space for them to explore what they can do for themselves, but more importantly, what they believe they need from their partner to help in this process. Assertive, honest communication techniques can be encouraged and explored so that the NOP can clearly communicate her needs to her partner.

One of the simplest, yet seems to be the most profound, things I say regularly with couples who choose to stay together is 'something good has to come out of something so bad'

This can help them work out what changes need to be made for themselves and for the relationship to work.

The partner who chooses to leave

Although leaving a partner who is convicted of a sex offence might seem like the obvious answer, it can still be extremely difficult to navigate. Telling the children, their wider family, and their friends who only yesterday all thought they were living happily together. I recall one lady saying it was like she had woken up after a nightmare; but sadly, the nightmare continues. For most there is a true grieving process, although their loved one is still alive (Duncan et al., 2022). Grieving is not always a linear process, however. In these cases, it commonly manifests in shock, disbelief, and even denial. This is often followed by fear and anger as the reality sets in. The NOP often will say they feel numb and find it difficult to understand how the world is continuing as normal around them. There is a complete feeling of overwhelm, sadness, loneliness, and despair. It's hardly surprising that non-offending partners suffer with anxiety and depression, despite them being innocent bystanders (Zilney, 2020).

Where there are children involved, it is extremely difficult to explain to them what their parent has done, the reason for leaving, or why the offender is leaving. Once again innocent bystanders are punished, in addition to the long-term damage that this does to the child's development and the possible impact on their future relationships (Webster, 2022).

If the community does find out what has happened, whether the couple stay together as a family or the NOP leaves, there is often prejudice towards the NOP and their children; whispers of 'she must have known'. Bullying in school is commonplace and other parents discourage their children from being friends with the offender's children, resulting in further alienation for them. I worked with one NOP who left her partner. She was well known in the community, so she had to change her name, her children's names, and move to a totally different part of the country, leaving her support network behind to start a completely new life elsewhere. When you take all of this into account, it gives a clearer understanding of why someone might stay with an offender, rather than leave. As a therapist, therefore, it is vital that you support the NOP to resource themselves, establish a support network and a safety plan for moving on.

In these circumstances, a therapist can play a crucial role in supporting the NOP in navigating their way through the various processes. Encouraging further support for the family and liaising with other services can be really helpful for the NOP, as you may be the only one who is truly empathic to their situation

Starting again

It might be that you are working with a NOP who has already left the offender but is now fearful of starting over again with a potential new partner. I worked with one lady who was ten years post-leaving her partner and was still struggling with considering starting over. Her trust of men in general was minimal, even those she felt close to. She showed heightened suspicion and was hypervigilant; it was as though she was completely stuck in her fight/flight response. She explained that she had been suspicious that her previous husband was having an affair; she was convinced that he was bringing the person to their home when she was out, as he seemed to be always encouraging her to go out with her friends. She was so suspicious that she installed a camera in their home and the next time she went out she recorded him. The shock was much worse than she could have ever imagined; he wasn't with another woman as she'd thought, he was being sexual with their family dog. It is these sorts of stories that make you understand why it would be so difficult to move on and attempt to start over with a new person. The memories and scars of the past can make it difficult to move on and consider a new relationship, with difficulties in trusting someone new, not only with yourself but potentially with their children too. Therapy can be particularly helpful at this time, giving someone the space to explore not only their fears but to encourage hopes and dreams of what could be, with the right person. Although it is important not to say 'don't worry it won't happen again' as no one can guarantee that. The therapeutic focus should be on self-reflection and healing. Therapy is a great place to do this, allowing a safe space to explore emotions, fears, potential triggers, and establishing boundaries in order to build a new relationship on trust and respect.

Whilst there are different modalities of therapy that can be helpful, it might also be worth considering Eye-Movement Desensitisation Reprocessing Therapy (EMDR); this can be particularly useful when someone is stuck and just doesn't feel or believe that they can move on from what has happened. It also does not require talking in detail about the trauma or experience, which can sometimes retrigger the traumatic memories, or the person just can't say the words because of the level of distress it causes them. There has been much research on EMDR therapy and it is recognised as an effective form of treatment for trauma and other disturbing experiences. Shapiro's (2001) Adaptive Information Processing model posits that EMDR therapy facilitates the accessing and processing of traumatic memories and other adverse life experience, to bring these to an adaptive resolution. After successful treatment with EMDR therapy, affective distress is relieved, negative beliefs are reformulated, and physiological arousal is reduced (EMDR.com).

The therapist: compassion fatigue

Although as therapists we are aware of compassion fatigue working in the field of counselling or therapy, this is particularly evident and evidenced when working with either sex offenders or the NOP (Figley, 2013; Pirelli, Forman, & Maloney, 2020). Even though you may not work with sex offenders directly, it can still have a similar impact, as you are not only hearing the stories of what the offender has done, but you are also hearing what the impact of those stories has been on the NOP, their children, and their wider lives. It is therefore crucial that therapists prioritise their own self-care. This should include regular supervision with someone skilled in this area of work, both individual and peer supervision can be particularly helpful. This gives you the opportunity to debrief, discuss difficult and complex cases, receive feedback that you are doing a good job, and that just knowing that you are not alone can be really beneficial, as it can be quite isolating work.

Continuing professional development is vital to keep up to date with the latest techniques and resources in this area of work, and in particular in relation to the NOP; this will help you feel more confident and competent in this field. This should also include understanding and training in the law in this area, particularly around confidentiality and safeguarding, which is paramount.

Self-care continuous professional development (CPD) can be useful too, as this gives you the opportunity to learn and practise new ideas to prevent compassion fatigue. Mindfulness and stress reduction techniques such as meditation and yoga can be really helpful in managing stress and being able to stay present for your client so as not to become emotional or feel overwhelmed in the session. Take regular breaks and try to engage in other activities that promote relaxation and fun! Keeping a good work/life balance is crucial in order to prevent burnout by limiting the number of clients you might see in a day and keeping a clear distinction between work and your personal life.

It is also important to keep your own relationships healthy as evidence demonstrates that therapists working in this field can start to question and distrust their own partners and those around them. This is where personal therapy can be particularly helpful; providing a safe place to share and process your inner feelings and emotions. It is also important to set boundaries as there is only so much you can do for your clients: limiting sessions by empowering them through information, guidance and signposting will help you 'share the load.'

Above all, please remember self-care, is not a luxury, it is essential.

Conclusion

In conclusion, the role of therapists working with the NOP of a person who has committed a sexual offence is both heart-wrenching yet rewarding. Whether the partner chooses to stay or chooses to leave in order to rebuild their lives and the lives of their children, the therapist will play a significant and crucial role in this process. The therapeutic journey is both challenging and complex both for the client and the therapist, but by offering empathic support and personalised interventions and a nurturing safe space to empower your client to take the journey of personal healing, they will be able to make an informed choice about their future. Regardless of the path they choose, the therapist will enable them to explore their feelings, express their emotions, and foster empowerment as they establish healthy boundaries and build resilience towards a greater emotional well-being.

References

Centre of Expertise on Child Sexual Abuse (2023) Managing risk and trauma after online sexual offending. csacentre.org.uk/research-resources/practice-resources/managing-risk-and-trauma-after-online-sexual-offending/.

Cahalane, H. & Duff, S.C. (2017) A qualitative analysis of nonoffending partners' experiences and perceptions following psychoeducational group intervention. *Journal of Sexual Aggression*, 24(1), 1–14.

Duncan, K., Wakeham, A., Winder, B., Armitage, R., Roberts, L., & Blagden, N. (2020) The experiences of non-offending partners of individuals who have committed sexual offences. Recommendations for practitioners and stakeholders. https://irep.ntu.ac.uk/id/eprint/41769/1/1392554_Winder.pdf.

Duncan, K., Wakeham, A., Winder, B., Blagden, N. & Armitage, R. (2022) 'Grieving someone who's still alive, that's hard': the experiences of non-offending partners of individuals who have sexually offended – an IPA study. *Journal of Sexual Aggression*, 28(3), 1–15. doi.org/10.1080/13552600.2021.2024611.

Figley, C. R. (2013) *Helping Traumatised Families*. Routledge.

Lytle, R., Bailey, D.J . S., & Bensel, T. (2017) We fought tooth and toenail: exploring the dynamics of romantic relationships among sex offenders who have desisted. *Criminal Justice Studies*, 30(2), 117–135. doi.org/10.1080/1478601x.2017.1299322.

Pirelli, G., Forman, D. L. & Maloney, K. (2020) Preventing vicarious trauma (VT), compassion fatigue (CF) and burnout (BO) in forensic mental health: Forensic psychology as an exemplar. *Professional Psychology; Research and Practice*, 51(5), 454–466. doi.org/10.1037/pro0000293.

Salter, M., Woodlock, D., & Jones, C. (2023) 'You Feel Like You Did Something So Wrong': Women's Experiences of a Loved One's Child Sexual Abuse Material Offending. *Violence Against Women*. doi.org/10.1177/10778012231208974.

Shapiro, F. (2001) *Eye Movement Desensitization and Reprocessing: basic principles, protocols and procedures*. 2nd ed. Guilford Press.

Smith, A. (2022) *Counselling Partners and Relatives of Individuals who have Sexually Offended: A Strengths-Focused Eclectic Approach*. Cadoc Publishing.

Steel, C. M. S., Newman, E., O'Rourke, S., & Quayle, E. (2022) Suicidal Ideation in Offenders Convicted of Child Sexual Exploitation Material Offences. *Behavioral Sciences & the Law*, 40(3). doi.org/10.1002/bsl.2560.

Stop it Now (2024) 'There is hope'. How protective parenting assessments and interventions protect children. Lucy Faithful Foundation. https://www.stopitnow.org.uk/home/media-centre/news/protective-parenting-blog/.

Webster, R. (2022) What's it like being the child of a sex offender? Russell Webster. https://www.russellwebster.com/whats-it-like-being-the-child-of-a-sex-offender.

Zilney, L. A. (2020) *Impacts of Sex Crime Laws on the Female Partners of Convicted Offenders*. Routledge.

Chapter 9

Working therapeutically with men who have sex with men who commit sexual offences

John Goss

Introduction

This chapter focuses specifically on working with men who identify as being gay, bisexual or men who have sex with men (MSM). This may include trans men, and quite often I will refer to men or gay men to encompass all those mentioned above. It will commence by examining the recent socio-political history of homosexuality in the UK, to give some context to the issue, because I will refer back to some of this throughout the chapter.

Although sex between men was decriminalised in 1967, it was only in 1990 that the World Health Organisation declared that being gay would no longer be deemed a 'mental illness', creating an age of consent of 21 years. In 1994, the Criminal Justice and Public Order Act reduced this to 18, and was eventually lowered to being 'equal' to heterosexuals, i.e. 16, in 2001. Section 28 of the Local Government Act 1988 prevented proper sex education for same sex male couples, to be repealed in 2000 (Scotland) and in England and Wales in 2003. It was only in 2005 that Civil Partnerships between same sex couples became legal with the introduction of the Civil Partnership Act (2004), and later marriage was permitted by The Marriage (Same Sex Couples) Act in 2013. It's important to reflect on this recent history because these events were not so long ago, and it is so easy to lose sight of these milestones.

The history of sex among MSM is varied and diverse. We still have generations of men among us where being gay would have been illegal. I am a firm believer that 'cottaging' (having sex in public toilets) and 'cruising' (sex in open areas, parks, fields, etc.) will have evolved from the prior restrictive legislation. The term 'cottaging' goes back to Victorian times when men would go to public baths, called cottages, to have casual sex. As being gay was illegal, this was the only way that MSM could meet others. Although society has become more open-minded in many respects regarding gay and pride activities, the legislation remains on the statute books: The Sexual Offences Act 2003 describes the act of engaging

DOI: 10.4324/9781003509103-11

in sexual activity in a public lavatory (section 71), and if prosecuted under this Act, a man would be placed on the Sexual Offender's Register.

Human immunodeficiency virus (HIV)

HIV remains an important global public health issue since it achieved epidemic proportions in the 1980s. Some MSM will have grown up through all this, in fear of catching HIV, although more recent pharmaceutical developments mean that taking one tablet a day (known as PREP) can prevent HIV transmission; not to forget that someone who is HIV+ and on medication, cannot pass the virus on. Of course, HIV does not just affect MSM, but it has historically been a large portion of MSM people who have been affected by HIV in the UK. When thinking about sexual offending, it's important to keep these historical issues in mind, because they may have influenced how MSM behave today.

Talking consent

More recently, dating apps like Grindr, Tinder, or Growlr (and some websites) have played a big part in the gay community, allowing the freedom for casual 'hook ups' at MSM's convenience, so there is less need to hook up in public toilets, putting themselves at risk of committing an offence. They also, however, in my view, blur the lines of consent in terms of what's agreed online and in person. Here we look at Michael, and issues around consent via dating Apps.

'Michael'

Michael was in his 30s and was a regular user of various dating Apps. He enjoyed the thrill of casual sex, and chatting to other men. He willingly shared pictures of himself, and they often shared pictures back. Often, Michael would invite men he chatted to back to his place for casual sex. They would chat about what they like on the dating App, and Michael would invite the person to his home for that to happen. One day, Michael is arrested for rape, after a complaint was made about him forcing sex on a man who had arrived to meet him for sex.

In the case study of Michael, he presented for therapy describing himself as 'shocked' that this has happened to him, and maintained that what he did was always consensual. In therapy, we explored the idea of consent and what this meant for Michael. One of the key things to crop up was that Michael felt that when he chatted on dating apps, consent was given during that chat (on the dating app). Therefore, when someone arrived for sex, he was forceful in 'getting it done' because in his mind, that was what had already been agreed (on the app). What Michael hadn't considered was that consent can be withdrawn, and consent or chat on a dating app should not be taken as consent in the real world.

The same situation applies for straight (heterosexual) men who have been eroticised by compulsively watching gay and trans pornography. They may feel they want to try it out, thinking their eroticism means that they may be covertly gay or bisexual, only to find that there is no 'turn on' when they hook up with someone in person. It's easy to chat on dating apps, and the ease of playing out a fantasy can be a real 'turn on' for some men, but that does not always mean that the erotic fantasy occurs in reality.

I have spoken to my own gay friends about consent, and it has been fascinating to hear their views, with opinions like 'if we chatted about it on the app, that means that consent was given'. Perhaps there's a sense or feeling that consent is something we agree to in messages on dating apps, but we must not forget that it can be withdrawn, or that someone might simply change their mind. Working with Michael was powerful, and a key part of our work was exploring consent, what it meant, how it is agreed, and him being able to accept that people can fantasise in chat online, but that does not always mean they want that reality in the same way.

For the next case study of Andrew, I draw us to a different piece of legislation: the Offences Against the Person Act 1861, which in the past has been used to prosecute someone who 'deliberately' transmitted HIV to another person.

'Andrew'

While working for a national helpline some years ago, I took a call from Andrew who had been chatting to another guy on a popular gay dating website (apps weren't around then). He called in to say that he had been chatting, and the person he had been chatting to had given him permission (consent) to go into his house and penetrate the awaiting sexual partner, anally, without using condoms.

In Andrew's case study, there is another classic example of 'consent' being agreed online and the act then happening. What Andrew did not disclose was his HIV status (he was HIV positive). At the time, medication was not as good as it is now, and messages about being *undetectable means untransmutable* (U=U) weren't around then. (U=U means that men with undetectable levels of HIV through prescribed medication is considered not to be able to transmit HIV.)

Andrew explained that in the hype (or excitement) of the online chat, he had got carried away and had not mentioned his HIV status. When invited over, Andrew took the opportunity and had sex as it had been agreed. It was only later, hence him calling the helpline, that he started to reflect on this, and panicking, sought our advice. After seeking opinions from colleagues, I was the one who called him back and advised him to encourage the recipient to seek Post Exposure Prophylaxis (PEP). This is a course of HIV treatment that if taken within 72 hours can help prevent HIV from taking effect in the body. I also had to advise him that he could (potentially) find himself in trouble, if he was seen not to notify any partners and was not using condoms.

Now I appreciate times have changed. People who are HIV+ positive can now enjoy condom-less sex if they are on treatment and have an undetectable viral load (VL) (U=U). We now also have PREP, a form of HIV medication that can be taken to prevent HIV. U=U messages and PREP weren't around when I took that call from Andrew that day. However, there are still fears in the community of being accused of being either reckless or intentional in the transmission of HIV (or other serious infections). There is a very good overview of prosecutions for HIV transmission produced by the Terence Higgins Trust (2010).

So, what has this got to do with sexual offending? Well, for me it is another example (all be it from some time ago) of how among MSM, consent can be seen to be agreed via messages and apps, and the perception then is that is consent applies in real life.

Chemsex

For some time now, 'Chemsex' has been an issue for MSM. A quick look on some dating apps will show people with taglines such as HnH (High and Horny) or 'Chilling' – another term, in my experience, where people might be doing 'chems'. Chemsex is used to describe a sexual behaviour, usually amongst men that have sex with men (MSM) under the influence of psychoactive drugs, primarily mephedrone (GHB), butyrolactone (GBL), and crystal methamphetamine. These drugs are often taken to facilitate sexual activities lasting several hours and, sometimes, days, with multiple sexual partners (Neves, 2021). Again, issues of consent arise during Chemsex because people do not necessarily know what they are doing, who they are doing it to or with, or where the boundaries of consent lie.

'Josh'

Josh was a teenager who had attended a sex party and while he was there, he had been injected with drugs and men had sex with him. His parents reported this to the police. While I have no full understanding of the case, it was believed he 'consented' when he attended the party, and had allowed someone to inject him. I am sure the trauma of that night will have stayed with him for a long time, and may still do, many years later.

The issue in Josh's case study is that when 'chems' are involved, the boundaries of consent are even more blurred. I have heard stories of people waking up to find someone is having sex with them; others talk of the constant lookout for someone to join in; and others speak of the time lost to chemsex. It can be days, weeks or years before some men seek support to come out of the cycle of it all.

'Alex'

Alex was a 30-year-old gay male living in London. He described having a good job and enjoyed being on the gay scene (including some of the cities sex clubs and saunas). He was offered 'G' (GHB) on one occasion and really enjoyed the sexual high that it gave him. Alex enjoyed the experience and the 'highs' and as a result started using dating apps to connect with people who might also be using chems. Chems and chemsex started to take more of a priority in his life, and as such his friendships and work took a back seat. During this time the relationship with his family was also impacted, although at the time they didn't quite realise the bigger picture of what's going on. The sex was a real high for Alex, and engaging in chems helped him feel more confident about himself and his body, and he felt like he was having harmless fun. One day Alex got a knock on the door; it was the police. Alex was arrested on suspicion of rape. Alex couldn't recall all the details of when the alleged offending happened, due to being so 'high' himself. This had a huge impact on him, and he found that using chems was his way of coping with situations.

Unfortunately, in Alex's case study, the therapeutic sessions ended before his case came to any sort of conclusion, so I am unable to share any outcome. However, he lost his job as a result, and other aspects of his life seemed to crumble away. He felt that he was too 'out of it' to truly know what had happened and struggled to remember any details. He had no past convictions or cautions, so this case was truly devastating for him.

What Alex's case does highlight though is how Chemsex had blurred the boundaries of consent. We don't truly know what happened on that occasion, and nor did Alex, but it had a massive impact on his life, and he always maintained he was too high to truly remember what had happened. The addictive side of chems, together with compulsive sex, often removes men from the 'here and now' due to the potentiated dopamine neural pathways (see Chapter 7).

Online offending

Most clients I work with as a therapist have offended online. This is true of my client and case study, who I shall name Sam.

'Sam'

Sam is in his late 50s and was arrested for possessing and sharing child sexual abuse material (CSAM). Sam was living with his husband at the time, who was also arrested (on suspicion) but later released without charge, as at that time, the police did not know which man had committed the offence, so they had to arrest them both until they could establish who was the alleged offender. No doubt, Sam's husband was not impressed and knew nothing about what had been going on. Nonetheless, he remained supportive of Sam throughout the investigation.

In Sam's case study, we explored his offending in therapy, and we looked back at his own sexual experiences from an early age. Sam grew up at a time when being gay was illegal; he saw homosexuality decriminalised and the various changes in the law that had happened since then. He had grown up in a world where being gay wasn't allowed; the law said so, and so did society. He felt that he did not fit in, and that getting a girlfriend and being married was seen as the 'normal' thing to do. He did not get married, but the idea that he was supposed to marry a woman and have children was a big influence on his life, creating a form of self-loathing; internalised homophobia. Similarly, the HIV scares of the 1980s also had a big impact on him, as he had seen his own friends die of AIDS-related illnesses. It is fair to say that Sam saw many legal and societal changes in his life, and later did marry someone (a man), with whom was generally happy.

In my therapy with Sam, we spent a lot of time exploring the impact of the legal aspects of Sam growing up when he did, and what impact these had on him on his self-esteem. Gay dating apps and websites did not exist when Sam was growing up and he certainly felt like he had 'missed out' on it all. He enjoyed chatting on websites with other men, and during the therapy sessions he disclosed he sometimes used drugs whilst online. Sam felt that when using chat rooms online he could connect with the social community he had missed out on when he was younger. He enjoyed the thrill of chatting to men all over the world and sharing pictures of himself with people he chatted to.

It was evident, and Sam agreed, that he often felt lonely. His husband worked during the day, whereas Sam had been made redundant after a long career. He could not necessarily see himself working again, and acknowledged that he was often bored when at home during the day. He took on fake personas online that he said he thought people would enjoy, and loved the online role-play challenges. Online chats would come and go, profiles that existed one day would have disappeared the next. Sharing pictures was fun and exciting, and coupled with the drugs, more exciting. Sam said that the pictures he received often did not mean much to him. He often felt desensitised to it all, but he did love the thrill of the chat and exchanging images. Chatting, he said, cured his boredom to some degree. It allowed him a means of escape, and sometimes felt he could connect with what he had missed out on.

During the investigation, the police revealed that Sam had been chatting to someone who was being monitored (not in the UK) and had engaged in swapping pictures and fantasy chat. The law enforcement in the other country informed the UK police, who then arrested him (and his husband, as mentioned above). Sam saw me for therapy for some time, and for a short while after his case concluded. He was handed a suspended sentence and was placed on the sex offender's register.

'Jack'

Jack was in his late 20s and described himself as a gay man. He was overweight and felt he did not fit into the gay scene. Sometimes he found other men to have been quite nasty to him on dating apps and believed that was due to his weight.

Jack didn't have a good relationship with his Dad, whom he described as often absent in his life. Jack came for therapy because he had been arrested for sharing pictures of himself and chatting to males younger than himself on social media. He disclosed during therapy that he had also used apps to share images of teenagers to other groups and found it quite a buzz in doing so. Jack said he did not feel attracted to people under the age of consent, but found an online community that accepted him, which spurred him on to continue.

In the case study of Jack, he and I explored in therapy his sense of attachment, particularly to his dad, of whom he did not have a high opinion. We also explored his sense of association (attachment) with the gay community. Jack felt isolated, and said that during the online conversations he was having, he felt accepted and he would admire younger gay guys (known as twinks), who were above the age of consent, but had a 'good body' and made him feel that is what he wanted to have been like. He said that this element for him was a sexual turn on, and seeing 'twinks' with a good physique made him feel better. He would often exchange pictures pretending to be younger than he was and found this exciting.

During this time, Jack expanded his so-called 'social network' of people who wanted to share pictures. He shared some he had received (consensually) from men, as well as pictures of himself. In turn he liked receiving pictures he had never seen before, and subsequently shared them out among his network too. It seemed that during this series of picture exchanges, Jack received (and shared) pictures of young men under 18 years. I discussed with Jack regarding receiving and sharing of CSAM, which he admitted to doing. He told me that getting images of that nature was initially a shock, but the shock element was also enjoyable, coupled with a sense of 'connection' that he did not feel he had with his own dad, and certainly did not feel he had within the gay community.

Conclusion

In this chapter, I have reviewed the historical process of homosexuality becoming legal in contemporary society. However, particularly for men whose lived experienced was to be criminalised for their sexual orientation, there is still a need in therapy to explore the contribution that this history makes, and any consequential internalised homophobia that may result. Similarly, there is still a fear amongst the gay community regarding the transmission of HIV, despite contemporary pharmaceutical medication being able to keep it in check. Modern-day communication within the gay community often takes place via social media and dating apps, but this process, as does the practice of chemsex, can blur the boundaries of providing consent for sexual encounters, as men may not realise that consent needs to be provided in the 'here and now'; that prior consent via social media is not sufficient. Consent whilst under the influence of alcohol or drugs (or both) is also not acceptable as a form of consent, and that men have the right to change their minds at any time. I finished by offering case studies of how men who were feeling excluded from the gay community can find themselves crossing the line into sexual offending.

References

Neves, S. (2021) *Compulsive Sexual Behaviours A Psycho-Sexual Treatment Guide for Clinicians*. Routledge.
Terence Higgins Trust (2010) Prosecutions for HIV transmission. /www.nat.org.uk/sites/default/files/onlineguides/May_2010_Prosecutions_for_HIV_Transmission.pdf.

Chapter 10

Prevention

Where the journey begins when
working with children

Terri Van-Leeson

Why work with children in this context?

Therapists working with forensic clients are seeing a significant increasing number of referrals of children unable to secure mainstream service support. Reasons for this are likely twofold: on the one hand it is common knowledge that child and adolescent mental health services (referred to as CAMHS) have become so stretched that waiting lists in some areas of the country are exceeding two years. Secondly many practitioners are anxious about their ability to work in this area, and feel ill-equipped about the type of skills required. Children require a different approach from working with adults, both in terms of content and process. When one introduces the subject of sex and sexual trauma, there is often a sense of avoidance and immediate anxiety provoked for many professionals.

This second reason is not new. Prior to CAMHS services becoming overwhelmed with demand across other areas of children's needs, it was not uncommon to see children who had been rejected by mainstream services, because they had themselves perpetrated sexually harmful behaviour toward other children. It is critical that these children are seen as equally deserving of service support, because leaving them to struggle can only mean one thing: they go on to develop deep rooted psychological and emotional problems and risk becoming criminalised in adulthood. It is time we begin to truly embrace the concept of prevention.

Prevention is the act of stopping something from happening or of stopping someone from doing something (Cambridge Dictionary, n.d.). How this translates into working with children is that it is essential to help the child address the source of *why* they are acting out in a sexualised way. To provide a shared understanding or language, I will use the term harmful sexual behaviour throughout this chapter. Sexualised behaviour also now incorporates internet-based activity.

DOI: 10.4324/9781003509103-12

Planning: the assessment of the child's needs

Firstly, we need to formulate (or speculate accurately, generating a set of reasons) why the child is acting out sexually. One needs to take a comprehensive background history of the child's life, up to the point of referral. We could call this the assessment or planning phase. This is essential before we start to work with a child, so that we are equipped with the essential knowledge about the child's life history, any attachment trauma, and whether they have been a victim of sexual abuse (and/or other abuse). We need to learn this information from the adult caregiver rather than asking the child for this type of information. We then also need to know what they have been doing that has caused concerns or triggered the need for other agencies to become involved in their lives, which could include the criminal justice system at some level.

Safeguarding

Work with children must be undertaken in a multi-agency way to always ensure child safeguarding. This means that other adults (*i.e.* parent, carers) and professionals (*i.e.* social worker, or support worker at school) outside of the therapeutic space know about the planned work, in terms of both the nature and purpose of the content. This protects the child, and it also protects you as the practitioner. This is a different way of working compared to adult work. It is transparent, collaborative, and supports the child outside of the therapeutic space. A meet-and-greet session is also essential initially, usually with the child's parent or carer (safe adult) present. It is essential that we do not role model children meeting strangers (you are as the practitioner) for the first time alone, whether it is face-to-face or online.

In terms of *process* this is where it is essential for the practitioner to work with the parent/foster-carer or lead professional if the child is in a local authority unit. Many children I have worked with have an assigned social worker who is centrally involved with the parent/caregiver from the outset, and throughout the work. However, on some occasions only the parent is involved. Whatever the child's social circumstances, it is always essential that a key adult is involved at all stages.

The reason for this is to safeguard the child in relation to you as the practitioner; for you to feel safeguarded too because some of the work may involve psycho-education about sex and sexual knowledge. Work undertaken with a child must be transparent at every stage, so that your practice is defensible and clear to other responsible adults about what the work comprises, what is planned, how the work unfolds, and what is concluded. It is essential to provide a short debrief after a session to an identified adult. These not only feed into the safeguarding aspect of the work, but also provide a means of support for the child outside of session time. For example, being able to provide a parent with the skill the child is going to try to use as an experiment to help him sleep better when feeling fearful, hypervigilant, or anxious.

To summarise, once a referral is received, this triggers a comprehensive assessment of the child's life history through information gathering with the parent/

caregiver and/or assigned social worker. From this we can determine the nature and extent of trauma the child has been subjected to, in parallel with what the child has been doing sexually that is causing concern or harm. An intervention plan can then be generated that specifically targets the child's profile. Sessions are planned, to commence with a 'meet-and-greet' with the parent/care-giver present. In some cases, the parent may continue to be present in sessions if this is helpful and/or necessary. The way de-brief post-sessions will occur is also identified from the outset.

Theory into practice: a trauma-informed approach

Work with all children needs to be underpinned by neuroscientific theory and child developmental theory. This is to ensure both the content and process of the work with each individual child and young person is optimised to be tailored to their specific needs, and their individualised sexual and developmental experiences.

It is important for the therapist to pitch the way one works with each child uniquely. For example, if you are to work with a child or young person who was sexually abused when they themselves were under the age of three years (the time when their own sexual trauma occurred) this means the child experienced their trauma during the pre-verbal phase of their early development; before their speech and language developed. The child will therefore not be able to 'talk' about, or use a verbal label to describe, what they experienced in their own body. This is because pre-verbal early life trauma events are stored in the brain and nervous system in a disorganised way. The child may instead be presenting as sad, confused, conflicted, and feeling shame. This can also likewise be the case for an adult abuse survivor who experienced sexual abuse during the pre-verbal phase of their development.

Critically, practitioners must never assume any child knows why they are doing what they are doing sexually in terms of the harmful sexual behaviour. This includes teenagers. It is easy to judge and analyse the sexualised behaviour through adult reasoning with adult knowledge. Instead, what the practitioner should do is put themselves in the shoes of the child, where the child is at developmentally, and importantly, what stage of development they were at when they experienced being sexually abused themselves. This is essential because it will help with the planning of the content and methods of the intervention.

A significant concept outlined in the trauma literature, and by Hudson-Allez (2011, 2020, 2024), is repetition compulsion, and it is important to have some understanding of this. This is relevant for children, particularly when they have been sexually abused during the pre-verbal phase of development. Repetition compulsion (i.e. the re-enacting of the abusive experience) according to Schwarz et al. 'arises because the brain's intrinsic healing mechanism senses the unresolved disturbance and recreates the contextual factors which may yet lead to a different outcome' (Schwarz et al., 2017, p. 38).

The trauma literature also helps us to consider the most appropriate methods to use with a child. For example, somatic methods that draw on the senses. Rather than relying on cognitive approaches (Marich, 2011) that ask of the child 'why did you do that?' or 'how did you feel?', somatic work is more appropriate. This is also often the case for adults with complex trauma suffered during childhood, but is essential for children.

Asking the child what they are feeling in their body or where they are feeling a sensation in their body can be more enabling for them to engage rather than trying to get them to describe a feeling in a sequence. Additionally, depending on the process for the individual child, other somatic methods including drawing, or playing an instrument, or moving around, can be the most helpful way of helping facilitate the child to express their trauma. Also, do not expect the child to make eye contact with the practitioner because their shame-activated response can be activated and make it difficult for them to relate to you. One also has to adjust one's expectation and understanding of eye contact with a child who is neurodiverse.

From expression of what trauma means for the child, the practitioner takes the lead in being clear, unambiguous, and directive in psychoeducation about the relevant areas. This is because a child should not be expected to 'know' or make links with complex concepts, and all concepts should also be illustrated visually or in some concrete style. For example, the use of feelings cards, feelings dice and card games can be an excellent way to work with a child. For younger children, use of a 'Worry Monster' also provides an excellent way of being able to work collaboratively with the child on complex concepts such as fear, anxiety, and other everyday problems that they are worrying about and do not know how to express this.

Trauma focused work directs the clinician to apply a phased approach when providing an intervention for a client. This can also be referred to as a three-phase approach, which is the safest, most ethical way to work with traumatised people. It is also essential to highlight that the trauma work, supporting the child to make sense of what has happened to them, is underpinned by the relevant phase 1 work. Phase 1 is the essential starting point that focuses on stabilisation and safety of the client. This will include helping the client to learn about what is happening to their brain and body, emotional regulation skills, grounding skills to help them re-focus back into the present, learning to use self-soothing skills, and a variety of distraction techniques. Breathing techniques are an essential component. Part of this phase of work also includes building a strong, secure and safe therapeutic alliance to provide the client with a 'safe base' to eventually work on their trauma, and to support them with building their strengths and resilience. In fact, aside of being clear and unambiguous telling the child that what happened to them was not their fault, the majority of the work with children may comprise equipping them with an array of core somatic self-soothing sensory skills to help them to be able to regulate strong negative emotional states, including shame.

It is also important to reaffirm the message to all children who have suffered sexual abuse themselves that it was not their fault. Indeed, many adult survivors I see need to be given this message in a clear, unambiguous way, repeating it frequently, because it can take a sexual abuse survivor years to be able to start to accept this, rather than continue with self-loathing and self-blaming.

Development of the sexual template

The neuroscience of the seven pre-programmed emotion circuits is instrumental in underpinning the work children (and adults). It is also now understood that attachment and emotional regulation are interlinked. Hudson-Allez (2011, 2020, 2024) has drawn on the neuroscientific theory and studies over the last 70 years to provide an explanation of how and why this theoretical area is critical to helping practitioners understand and work with children and adults who have suffered sexual trauma.

Hudson-Allez outlines how we are born with seven pre-programmed emotional brain circuits which are designed to protect us as a vulnerable infant from harm and enhance our survival. These circuits are part of our neurobiological wiring. The seventh, the LUST circuit (after Panksepp, 1998), is for sexual arousal and satisfaction and is used to motivate reproduction of the human species. For children and young people who have experienced sexual abuse, the LUST circuit is activated too early. Hudson-Allez refers to this as the vandalisation of the sexual template. This circuit is only meant to be activated between the ages of five and nine with developmental changes that drive same age-appropriate sexual play. The sexual template developed by our sexual experiences prepares us for the onset of puberty, which is around ten years old and the subsequent sexual play and adolescent sexual experimentation. The sexual template provides the internal working model of how a child will behave sexually when they become an adult. Sexual abuse (including witnessing abuse and seeing pornography) in childhood can have a negative effect on adult sexual behaviour because it changes the way the sexual template develops. This can cause some people to develop sexual behaviours that society may view as distasteful, unusual, or abnormal. If the LUST circuit is activated too soon, the child cannot understand or deal with this LUST activation and the associated thoughts and feelings it starts activating. This is key to understanding how to work with children in my view. This can explain why some children who have experienced early sexualisation will start sexual activity with others at a young age.

Two case studies

Firstly, let us consider children who have experienced a known sexual abuse trauma history. These children commonly present with trauma re-enactment sexualised behaviour. Enacting what they had experienced and not being able to say why they are doing what they are doing, despite feeling bad about it and being told that it is 'wrong' for them to act in this way with other siblings or friends. This is also referred to as repetition compulsion being exhibited by the child (see below).

'Jacob'

Jacob is a six-year-old boy who was referred for support work follow-ing him engaging in an act of sexually inappropriate behaviour. Refer-ral was initiated through a social worker. A three-way consultation meeting took place between the social worker, mother/parent, and the practitioner. The purpose of this was to initially screen the referral, to make sense of what has happened and consider if we could offer him ap-propriate work to meet his needs. Key information gathered from the initial consultation was that Jacob had a disclosed sexual abuse trauma history that had been perpetrated toward him by his biological father with whom he was no longer in contact. Jacob was sexually abused during the pre-verbal phase of his own development (estimated to have been when he was two to four years old). When he was four years old, the boy described to his mother [about the abuse] what his father used to do to him when they were alone. His parents had separated when he was around two years old. The child's mother disclosed this infor-mation to the Police and safeguarding measures were initiated. When Jacob was four and a half years old, he had been offered play therapy for a time-bounded period by one of the allied health-related child services to help him process what had happened to him. He had engaged in art therapy for a short period, although no other information was available about this intervention. When Jacob was six years old, he enacted his sexual abuse trauma out on a friend who was of a similar age. This child disclosed the game they had played with Jacob to their parent, and con-sequently Jacob's sexually harmful behaviour came to the attention of the parent and to social services. Mainstream services would then no longer offer Jacob support therapies because he himself had in effect, become a perpetrator.

In Jacob's case study, the referral to StopSO was considered appropriate and therapeutic intervention work was offered to him. A transparent, joined-up way of working was agreed through a plan with the social worker, mother, and the school head teacher. This included practical factors, such as the mother always being pre-sent in a session, or a nominated (same) school support worker. Sessions needed to take place outside of the home environment. School became the focus of where the sessions took place online via Teams. Following each session, a debrief took place with the mother. This was to summarise how the child had presented in the session, what had been covered, and what to look out for in him and his emotional coping during the ensuing period after the session. Ways of reinforcing skills talked about in session were also explained to the mother, so she could help her son between sessions to try out some of the skills when he was unable to sleep, felt hypervigilant, anxious, or angry.

Therapy intervention plan

What follows is an outline of both the *process* and the *content* of the work with this child.

Process

Jacob engaged in a total of 25 sessions. During each session, his mother or the same nominated school support worker were present to support him. The presence of another responsible adult was important because he was a child under the age of ten years and sexual issues may be discussed with him if he raised them. We considered it important to ensure transparent practice which also amounted to ongoing effective safeguarding for him.

The *process* of the work with Jacob began by having a meet-and-greet session with him and his mother. One of the therapy intervention goals was to work on establishing a strong, safe working alliance with Jacob to become a 'safe adult' in his life; someone he could identify with who also talks with his safe adult/mother attachment, and someone he knows who also understood his history. He was already equipped with the knowledge of what had happened to him in his life and what he had been doing which had got him into trouble. Relevant for the process was the need to create a safe space for him, so that he knew he did not have to describe or explain himself to the practitioner. Instead, Jacob could come to his session knowing that the practitioner was not going to interrogate him by asking lots of shaming questions. Jacob had already previously been spoken to by the police and had found it distressing. He had received the 'knock' with uniformed police at his home.

The therapeutic approach in Jacob's case may differ from working with an adult whereby some practitioners use the first couple of sessions assessing the needs of the client by taking a detailed history. The meet-and-greet session became the opportunity for me to introduce myself to Jacob and reassure him. I told him that I knew his mother and we had been speaking to each other to start to think about how we could help him with some of his difficulties. Lots of reassurance was given during the meet and greet session, to ensure he realised he did not have to talk to me unless he wanted to. I told him how brave I thought he was, and that I also knew that things had happened to him in his life that he felt sad and confused about and I wanted to be able to help him; that I also knew there were things that he had done in his life that he felt confused and worried about and that I also wanted to help him with these things too. Jacob responded well to this and kept referring to his history as 'the stuff', to which I thereafter used as his language going forward.

In terms of the *process* element of Jacob's case, I was consistent across all sessions with Jacob. At the start of each session, I would explain I was pleased to see him, that he was brave for coming to the session. I would then ask him how he had been coping since our previous session, referring to one or two of the skills we had been talking about. After the initial sessions had taken place on psychoeducation of feelings and what they were experienced like and where they were in his body, I would always ask him about how he was feeling with the feelings cards and the feelings dice. At the close of the sessions we agreed together on what sort of experiment he could do to help him sleep better, and to manage his angry feelings. He embraced the idea of being a little scientist doing experiments between sessions, such as putting his music on low when trying to get to sleep to distract and sooth his 'head' (intrusive thoughts).

Content

The first several sessions engaged Jacob with learning about feelings, what they are and what they look like in his body. This psychoeducation phase was essential. Many children will not have an emotion vocabulary or language to use to be able to identify and describe how they are feeling. This was particularly relevant for Jacob who was feeling sad, confused, and frightened his abuser might walk into his house. He was unable to sleep. He also experienced strong negative emotional states of anger but did not know why or where these feelings were coming from.

Session 2 with Jacob began with learning about the 'worry monster'. It was pre-arranged for his mother to purchase a worry monster and a pack of emotion cards to bring to the session. I, as the practitioner, had my own worry monster and emotions cards so that we could both hold our worry monsters and begin to learn about what the worry monster could do to help us. I asked Jacob where worry would be in his body. He told me worry is in his tummy when he has done something wrong and is worried that he will be told off.

The worry monster meant we were able to work with what are complex concepts to a child. It meant we could start working on emotions and feelings in a way that was conceptually and somatically meaningful for Jacob to relate to. The worry monster therefore became a feature throughout the work. Jacob would write on a piece of paper, or draw a picture of his 'worry', place it in the worry monster's mouth and zip it up to get rid of it. His mother would then check the worry monster, and remove the paper. This way we could identify what some of the ongoing issues were that Jacob was trying to process. The physical removal of the 'worry' from the monster daily or whenever necessary was also a concrete way of teaching Jacob that he could share his worry and that this is a healthy thing to do, rather than suppress and not talk about things that were troubling him. I could then also ensure session time helped Jacob to be able to identify what some of his feelings were, using drawing, the emotion dice, and cards; he particularly liked the cards, and worked on them in session time.

Sessions included facilitating Jacob learning to talk about his feelings on a number of key issues through identifying in his body where a feeling was. Jacob learnt the skill of 'urge surfing' to be able to recognise when he had an angry feeling, that a feeling can build and build to the point, just like a wave, where it eventually peaks and calms down. Jacob became very adept at describing his waves of feelings and sometimes he described 'tsunamis' of feelings that were in lots of parts of his body and his head.

Other aspects of the psychoeducative work included skills-learning and practice, with the support of his mother between sessions. These were essentially helpful emotion regulation skills and distress tolerance skills. Examples being listening to music (low volume) at bed time that Jacob liked that would help him to counter intrusive thoughts; switching on when feeling tense, angry or anxious; having a 'calm down' space in the house he could go to and self-talk. He said, 'I am counting to ten and although I am feeling angry right now, I know the wave will crash and go away'. He used the word 'comfort' to help him to self-sooth and he identified and used a particular soft toy that became his grounding, soothing object that was very powerful for him. He was permitted to take this item to school.

From building on helping Jacob to be able to develop emotional regulation skills, we were then able to use these to support him to talk about his own trauma if he chose to do so, which was always at the forefront of his mind. It was important that I did not shy away from Jacob's trauma because of his young age. On the contrary for this child, he wanted to talk and he wanted to understand why he felt so confused, angry, sad, and frightened, sometimes all at the same time. It is important, though, to recognise that other children present differently and so the approach and content covered should go at the pace of the child, and where the child wishes to go.

To summarise my work with Jacob, some of the practical aspects of the content were: using emotions cards, emotion dice, a worry monster, drawing pictures, having a self-soothing toy that became a very significant feature, having a calm-down space, using music, playing games, and swimming, and talking about things he was good at doing in school. Jacob also enacted some aspects of what he does to cope, for example moving his body around the room space and pretending he was doing something at home that he enjoys. He did this naturally and so I, as the practitioner, went with how he chose to work.

The other essential feature of this work with children is that the practitioner needs to be clear, calm, and provide understandable explanations. Explanations should never be ambiguous and the practitioner should not expect the child to interpret meanings. The child needs clarity, guidance, and reassurance; explaining that the sexual abuse the child has suffered is not their fault. By explaining in this case, the sexual abuse then gets trapped in the brain, and as the brain is trying hard to make sense of what has happened in their body, they might act it out on someone else and then afterwards feel very bad about what they have done (repetition compulsion).

The second case study I will discuss, that of Andrew, will be an example of an increasing number of referrals we are seeing with children who have no known sexual abuse history, who have a pre-existing diagnosis of an autism spectrum disorder and who are either referred through the services for having been investigated by the police for inappropriate internet usage or have been exhibiting sexually inappropriate behaviour that a parent or school have become concerned about (see also Chapter 11 discussing neurodiversity).

'Andrew'

Andrew is a 15-year-old boy who had a pre-existing diagnosis of high functioning autism spectrum disorder (hereafter referred to as hfASD). He had been accessing indecent images of children (CSAM) material on the internet. He was initially arrested by the police and placed under investigation. He and his parents worked with the children's services, the youth offending service, and the police. The outcome resulted in Andrew not being charged. Instead, a safety plan was agreed with his parents on internet-enabled devices and his supervised access at home and school, in parallel with specialist intervention work to help him address his behaviour. An initial consultation took place with Andrew's mother and social worker. The assessment, or history-taking phase, was undertaken at this stage rather than with Jacob, the purpose being to generate a formulation and plan the intervention without needing to ask Andrew lots of shaming questions. Andrew, although 15 years old, was operating at a lower chronological age estimated to be around ten years old.

Therapy intervention plan

Process and content are outlined to demonstrate the areas of similarity, but principally differences, in this case study compared to that of Jacob.

Process

This began with Andrew and his mother being present for the meet-and-greet session. It had been agreed that all sessions were to take place at the family home in the study after school at the same time every week to create a routine for him to get used to.

Andrew was anxious and worried, and did not want to look at the screen. As the practitioner, I was flexible in how he presented so went with this, instead talking to him and his mum about how brave he was to even be in the room; that he did not have to come and look at the screen if he did not want to and that was okay; that he could hear and listen to me was more than good enough. In terms of the content of this first session, I explained that I work with young people who have done something that has got them into trouble with the police and we have been able to help them to learn how to avoid getting into any further trouble. Andrew's mum also kept reiterating that nothing he said would shock me, and that he would be able to talk to me and ask me anything he wanted about sex and sexual development.

Andrew completed 26 sessions. The process aspect of the work required me to focus more extensively on building up a trusting relationship with him during the first several sessions, before we could start to cover the content of the work in any detail. This was because Andrew presented for the first several sessions as fearful and anxious. He was terrified of going to prison, and held a strong belief that he would have to go to prison. Therefore, the content of the initial sessions involved explaining the process of what the police and the services had done, and that he was not going to prison. I had attended a case conference at which the police had been involved in the decision-making to agree no charges with the Crown Prosecution Service. I explained I was someone experienced in this work, and how the police and the courts work. It had been agreed by everyone at the 'meeting' about him that provided he was able to learn about why looking at CSAM was breaking the law and harmful, and he made a commitment to avoid doing it again, he would not need to worry about going to prison. Explanations had to be clear, concrete, in unambiguous language, and repeated several times. Eventually Andrew began to engage and felt okay, or less anxious about seeing me each session. By Session 4 he was always sitting closely looking into the screen.

Andrew told me that he had wanted to learn about sex and so had used the internet to find things out. He had looked at lots of different sites to do with sex and sexy things and had eventually gone on to access CSAM viewing naked children. Andrew explained he had been masturbating to some of these images he had seen. I, as the practitioner, asked him about the images that he had become aroused by. I asked him how we would refer to these images and he decided they were to be called the 'bad' images. We used his language for the duration of the work on his sexual functioning.

Content

The content of the work included psychoeducation about sexual development of the human body (and so his body), puberty, why we get sexual feelings, how we know when we are sexually aroused, what it looks like in our body and what we can do to gain sexual pleasure and release in a safe, legal way. Consent, the legal age for having sexual activity with another person, and other essential aspects of education about the law and sex (*i.e.* sexting) were also covered with Andrew. Once we got into the work, Andrew began to ask more questions and his confidence grew significantly. Andrew began to call me 'Terrigle', as opposed to Google, and this seemed to allow him to be able to ask me whatever he wanted without being as embarrassed and ashamed when comparted to the initial part of the work.

To summarise, other areas of content covered with Andrew were how we develop our sexual template, sexual interests, and sexual arousal to certain images or thoughts. Andrew called this the 'sex programme' in the body, because he found it more helpful to think about the body and the brain as being programmed to be able to do certain things. We adapted the language for complex concepts and it worked well to facilitate his learning of complex concepts around sexual arousal, sexual priming, and sexually primed neuropathways in the brain so that we could then work on directed masturbation techniques (a form of behavioural modification work, although this type of language was not used with him).

A final point to make from working with Andrew is we should never underestimate how little a teenage child knows about their sexual development, even when they have had some level of sex education, or a previous intervention. This had been the case for Andrew who had been told about masturbation as an acceptable behaviour to do alone in the privacy of his own room, yet Andrew still did not know what masturbation was, nor how to engage with this behaviour in a safe, healthy way.

Conclusion

Working with children requires being informed by an understanding of child developmental theory and how this applies to practice. It requires an ability to be responsive, flexible, and able to work at the pace of each individual child. Being clear, directive, and reassuring in explanations about not being to blame are also key aspects of the work, tempered skilfully with separating out what the child has gone on to re-enact as undesirable behaviours, which we want to help the child not to repeat in future.

Emotional regulation work and psychoeducation across key areas (i.e. emotions, trauma, and sex) should be delivered in somatic, concrete, sensitive, and unambiguous ways. When we start engaging meaningfully with where a child's needs are presenting at the time following an episode of harmful sexual behaviour or worrying sexual activity that has come to the attention of the police or allied public services, we are truly embracing a culture of prevention. Embracing this cultural shift will allow practitioners to untangle and address the cause of the unhealthy sexualised behaviour before established patterns form. By doing so we equip these children with the necessary knowledge and skills to be able to repair their developing sexual template. They can go on to develop healthy arousal pathways in the right way and in the right context as they grow into adulthood.

References

Cambridge Dictionary (n.d.) https://dictionary.cambridge.org/.

Hudson-Allez, G. (2011) *Infant Losses, Adult Searches. A neural and developmental perspective on psychopathology and sexual offending.* 2nd ed. Karnac.

Hudson-Allez, G. (2020) Attachments and Neuroscience. Understanding the role of brain development in children. Online training for College of Sexual and Relationship Therapists, 17 September 2020.

Hudson-Allez, G. (2024) *A Trauma-Informed Understanding of Online Offending: Adult Losses from Adolescent Searches.* Routledge.

Marich, J. (2011) *EMDR Made Simple: 4 Approaches to Using EMDR with Every Client.* Premier Publishing and Media.

Panksepp, J. (1998) *Affective Neuroscience. The Foundations of Human and Animal Emotions.* Oxford University Press.

Schwarz, L., Corrigan, F., Hull, A., & Raju, R. (2017) *The Comprehensive Resource Model: Effective Techniques for the Hearing of Complex Trauma.* Routledge.

Chapter 11

'How did I get into this? How could I have been so stupid?' The high-functioning neurodivergent client

Clare S. Allely

Potential innate vulnerabilities

Clients with undiagnosed high functioning autistic spectrum disorder (hfASD) are an over-representative proportion of clients getting the knock for online offences, most commonly viewing child sexual abuse material, extreme pornography, or sexual chat with 'friends' through social media who prove to be under the age of 18 years. For the purposes of this chapter and within a forensic setting, the author has chosen to use the terminology of 'an individual with autism' or 'an individual with an autistic disorder'. The reason for this is to be clear within the criminal justice system that barristers and judges understand that the person is impaired by this, with co-existing mental health issues, like life-long anxiety and/ or depression, rather than having their autism dismissed on the grounds that we are all on the spectrum somewhere. In this way, I am protecting the integrity of the diagnosis.

Therapists working with individuals with diagnosed hfASD, or missed diagnosed hfASD (Eaton, 2023), need to recognise and understand that they have some potential innate vulnerabilities if they have been charged with the viewing of child sexual abuse material (CSAM). Having an interest in CSAM is not an anticipated characteristic in individuals with hfASD (Attwood, Hénault, & Dubin, 2014; Mahoney, 2021). However, the literature (e.g., Freckelton, 2011, 2013; Allely & Dubin, 2018; Allely, Kennedy, & Warren, 2019; Allely, 2020, 2022) highlights that there is a range of possible innate vulnerabilities in some individuals with ASD who are charged with the viewing of CSAM. Some of these possible innate vulnerabilities include:

- Counterfeit deviance
- Social immaturity
- Being unaware of any moral or legal boundaries
- Literal and dogmatic thinking
- Impaired theory-of-mind (ToM)
- Impaired ability to correctly guess the age of victims in CSAM

DOI: 10.4324/9781003509103-13

- Impaired ability to recognise negative facial expressions of victims in CSAM
- The importance of considering the ritualistic nature of collecting CSAM in individuals with hfASD and the coexisting obsessive-compulsive behaviour

Each of these will now be described in detail in turn below.

Counterfeit deviance

The term 'counterfeit deviance' was first coined by Dorothy Griffiths (see Griffiths et al., 2013). The viewing of sexual material which is extreme in nature is not always predictive of deviant sexuality. Instead, it may be considered counterfeit deviance as opposed to deviant sexuality (Mahoney, 2017). Counterfeit deviance refers to a misperception of the intention of individual's motivations, which are perceived as sexual or deviant when they are not. Mark Mahoney, an attorney who works in the United States, who has defended a significant number of individuals with ASD on charges of possession of CSAM, incorporates the concept of counterfeit deviance in understanding what appears on the surface to be deviant behaviour but the individual 'lacks the culpable mental state or blameworthiness which would normally attend such actions by persons who are typically developed' (Mahoney, 2017, p. 19). What appears to be malicious intent is often due to the social misunderstandings of the individual with ASD (Kumar et.al., 2017).

Social maturity

The social and behavioural impairments that characterise hfASD may have a negative impact on sexual development (Sevlever, Roth, & Gillis, 2013). There are a variety of reasons for this. For instance, the adolescent with ASD may not have positive peer support and relationships. They may also receive limited sexual education from adults, both at home and school (Brown-LaVoie, Viecili, & Weiss, 2014). Some individuals with ASD may use the internet to get information about sex and sexual relationships or to satisfy sexual needs, which they are not able to do with to with peers and or friends (Dubin, Hénault, & Attwood, 2014). Studies have also found that young people with ASD are more likely to use media and pornography as a means of obtaining knowledge about sex compared to their typically developing peers and equally may rely on television rather than their parents, teachers, and peers for education or information on sexual issues (Pecora, Mesibov, & Stokes, 2016). When using the internet to seek information about sex and sexual relationships or to satisfy sexual needs, some young people with ASD may focus on circumscribed fields of interest and can quickly become intensely attached leading them to download and look at/watch more pornography or CSAM (Mahoney, 2017). When an individual with ASD has a circumscribed interest, their searches online regarding this interest will not be limited to a superficial internet search as it typically would with a neurotypical individual. Their searches on their circumscribed interest will be obsessive and extensive which may increase the risk of them coming across CSAM (Tantam, 2000).

The online world can be particularly appealing to individuals with ASD as it is easier to predict, logical, and does not involve emotional communication; it is a safe space (Mahoney, 2009). It is a misconception that when individuals with ASD spend a lot of time online that they are antisocial. The online world does not present the same challenges as face-to-face interactions. For instance, with computer-mediated interaction (CMI), they can take their time to process and respond to questions or what the other person is saying. CMI does not have the distracting or overwhelming number of stimuli that occur during face-to-face interactions such as facial expressions, different tones of voice, non-verbal body language, background noise, etc.

An individual with ASD can have an intelligence level which is above average while their social maturity can be well below average and closer to that of someone much younger. This often means that the individual prefers and feels safer when with younger people. They are at a similar emotional or social level to them (Cutler, 2013). It is also important to emphasise that neurodivergent clients are not more likely to commit sexual offences. However, anecdotally, they do seem more likely to fall down the rabbit hole traps that computer algorithms encourage. Also, images posted in chat rooms about computer games or topics which are appealing to many individuals with ASD, such as Japanese style animations (anime, hentai, manga); 'furries'; 'My Little Pony,' etc, may lead them to search for these things and suggestions are made in the computer algorithms that can be very quickly disturbing content.

Unaware of any moral or legal boundaries

Due to social isolation and sexual naivety, some individuals with ASD, may be completely unaware of any ethical, moral or legal boundaries with regards to CSAM. 'The lack of sociosexual knowledge is always the major issue' (Hénault, 2014, as cited in Mahoney, 2021). It is common for individuals with ASD to have diverse sexual interests, unrestrained by social and legal taboos. As an example, they may search for and view 'hentai' which are pornographic versions of anime on Google. It is useful to note here that, anecdotally, it is well known that an interest in anime is relatively common in individuals with ASD (e.g., see https://www.youtube.com/watch?v=30nfka8J8Y0; https://reelrundown.com/animation/Why-Are-Autistic-People-Drawn-to-Anime). One of the key explanations for why some individuals with ASD find anime so appealing is the fact that the characters have relatively simple and easy to read exaggerated facial expressions. What is common in individuals with ASD is an impaired ability to identify and recognise other people's facial expressions (particularly negative facial expressions such as fear, sadness, and distress). This is a well-established empirical finding in the academic literature. Anime, because the facial expression (and the faces themselves) are much simpler (e.g., giant eyes) and exaggerated (in terms of both the features of the face and the emotional expressions), are much easier to read and understand and, therefore, more relatable to some individuals with ASD. Given that an individual with ASD would find these images appealing for the above reasons, it is not surprising that they would gravitate towards the same images which are sexualised in nature both for sexual gratification and for learning and exploring sexual things. Many adolescents and young adults with ASD tend to be more emotionally or socially immature (both sexually and otherwise) when compared to their counterparts without a diagnosis of ASD.

Literal thinking

Many individuals with ASD who are charged with viewing CSAM very commonly state that one of the reasons they failed to recognise that what they were doing was illegal was that they were able to access the material freely online. The mere presence of CSAM on the internet gives the message of legality of the material to some individuals with ASD due to their literal black-and-white view of the world (Mesibov & Sreckovic, 2017). What they have been told about illegal pornography or CSAM cannot apply to what they are viewing on their computer because how bad can the imagery actually be if it accessible on the internet free of charge? (Sugrue, 2017). Sugrue also highlights that difficulties with central coherence and fluid reasoning which is common in ASD contribute to this thought processing, leading to the individual to have difficulty fully understanding the illegality of their behaviour or the consequences of what they are doing. Specifically:

> people on the spectrum process information differently to neurotypical. They can be told something, hear something, or read something, but without constant repetition and numerous examples that expand the range of applications for newly learned information, there is often a flawed understanding.
>
> (Sugrue, 2017, p. 119)

Also, they may see images and videos of young children made to look older in mainstream media, magazines, television, etc. They may not necessarily understand that looking at similar material on their computer in the privacy of their home would be inappropriate or illegal (Allely, 2022).

Impaired theory-of-mind (ToM)

It is common for individuals with ASD to be impaired in tasks involving theory-of-mind (ToM). ToM refers to an individual's ability to understand that other people have different thoughts, desires, beliefs, and intentions from them. The broader contextual issues relating to the CSAM may be something that the individual with ASD is completely unaware of. For instance, where and how they got the CSAM, who else may be able to access the material (Mesibov & Sreckovic, 2017) due to their impaired ToM. Individuals with ASD tend to have greater difficulty appreciating and understanding the perspective, thoughts, and experiences of other people when compared to neurotypical individuals. Individuals with ASD may find it more difficult to appreciate the perspective and experiences of the minors in the images or video they are looking at (Attwood, Hénault, & Dubin, 2014). There may be a 'sense of emotional detachment' while looking at CSAM on their computer. Additionally, features of impaired executive functioning can cause individuals with ASD who look at CSAM to have impaired ability to appreciate the broader perspective of their behaviours and the consequences to themselves (Attwood, Evans, & Lesko, 2014).

Impaired ability to correctly guess age

An impaired ability to accurately estimate the age of the individuals in the material they are looking at on the internet is another reason why some individuals with ASD may view CSAM without appreciating the illegality of their actions. It is important to consider this impaired ability to correctly guess age and the presence of blurred boundaries between adult and child given that the age of the victims in the material directly impacts on the legalist and severity of the offence (Mahoney, 2009). This difficulty can be exacerbated by the media which is saturated with content where the boundary between what is an adult and a minor are made intentionally blurry. Young teenage models are made to look much older (e.g., with the way they are dressed and the type of make-up) and older models are made to look much younger. For some individuals with ASD, these types of images can be particularly confusing to identify as being illegal (Mesibov & Sreckovic, 2017).

Impaired ability to recognise negative facial expressions in CSAM

Empirical literature has long found that individuals with ASD are, overall, impaired in their ability to recognise facial expressions (Uljarevic & Hamilton, 2013). They are particularly impaired in their ability to recognise negative emotional expressions such as fear, distress, anger, etc. (de la Cuesta, 2010). This impairment has obvious implications when such individuals are engaging with CSAM.

The ritualistic nature of collecting CSAM in individuals with ASD

As with any other type of preoccupation and interest, the desire for CSAM material can be significantly excessive and compulsive. In cases of individuals with ASD who have been charged with CSAM related offending, it is common for there to be substantially large collections as a result of the ritualistic and compulsive nature that coexists with ASD, with hundreds of files downloaded on their computer/ devices, many of which have not been accessed and remain unopened (Mesibov & Sreckovic, 2017). In many cases of individuals with ASD who are charged with possession of CSAM, there is evidence of extensive categorisation of the images/ videos. Take the following example of a male with a diagnosis of ASD who we will call Mr A.

'Mr A'

Mr A said that he did not set out with any aim but would just go into a variety of websites (e.g., X (Twitter), Instagram, etc) to see what he could collect; sometimes his searches would also be carried out on foreign sites. He would categorise the images or videos according to a range of features such as: eye colour; hair colour; skin colour; age, etc. He would often have the same image in more than one folder because it fell into more than one category. When Mr. A was visiting the different websites where he would collect his material, he would initially put all material into one folder which he would categorise at a later time. He reported spending hours organising the material. He also would engage in a similar collecting and categorisation process with images of animals. He also collected images from movies and would have subcategories for each character. Characters from the movies were both male and female. He would give the folders names according to the character he was collecting the images of. This was something he did for both the 'real-life' movies/films and the cartoon or anime characters. He said he would find it very frustrating that there were no details about the exact ages of the individuals in the material to enable him to categorise them accurately. He was sometimes forced to estimate the age and put them into folders such as individuals aged ten to 15, 16 to 19 years, 20 to 30 years, etc.

In Mr. A's case study, his frustration at being unable to get exact ages for the purposes of detailed, specific and accurate age categorisation is consistent with ASD and his ritualic, compulsive need to collect and categorise the material.

Although not the case for all individuals with ASD, 'sexuality can sometimes take on an added dimension and become a true obsession' (Hénault, 2014, p. 202). There is relatively little empirical research investigating this. However, based on her clinical experience, Dr Isabelle Hénault (a psychologist from the University of Québec at Montréal, Canada) has found this in a number of individuals with ASD. Obsessions are uncontrollable desires which are typically coupled with anxiety. When sexuality becomes the circumscribed interest of the individual with ASD, it becomes the only thing in their life which gives them stimulation to the detriment of other areas of their life such as social and occupational functioning (Hénault, 2014).

Alexithymia

Many individuals with ASD experience a lack of emotional awareness or an impaired ability or difficulty in identifying and describing feelings and in being able to distinguish feelings from the bodily sensations of emotional arousal. Such difficulty is typically referred to as alexithymia which is where the individual has an inability to recognise or describe one's own thoughts and emotions (Bird & Cook, 2013). Alexithymia is a multidimensional construct which consists of three components. These are:

(1) Difficulty identifying one's own feelings (DIF)
(2) Difficulty describing feelings (DDF)
(3) An externally orientated thinking style (EOT) whereby one tends to not focus their attention on their emotions.

Individuals with high levels of alexithymia have difficulty focusing attention on their emotional states (EOT) as well as experiencing a difficulty in being able to accurately appraise what those states are (DIF, DDF) (Preece et al., 2017). Research indicates that co-occurring alexithymia is highly prevalent in individuals with ASD and it has even been suggested that it underlies some socio-emotional difficulties which were previously attributed to ASD. Research has found that between 40% and 65% of the ASD population are alexithymic (see the review and meta-analysis in Kinnaird, Stewart, & Tchanturia, 2019). Studies suggest that emotion processing difficulties in ASD are driven by alexithymia (e.g., Cook et al., 2013). There are a number of measures for alexithymia, such as the Toronto Alexithymia Scale (TAS; Bagby, Parker, & Taylor, 1994).

Nick Dubin

Nick Dubin, at the age of 33 years, was arrested for the possession of CSAM in the United States. In his book, which he co-authored with Isabelle Hénault and Tony Attwood, Nick gives an in-depth personal account of his experiences of the criminal justice system as well as his experience growing up (Dubin, Hénault, & Attwood, 2014). In 2004, he was formally diagnosed with Asperger's Syndrome (now known as ASD). It is important to highlight that to think of someone with ASD as being on a spectrum (ranging from severely impaired to mildly impaired) can be misleading. Rather, it is more appropriate and accurate to consider each person with ASD separately and their particular profile of strengths and weaknesses; in other words, that individual's particular variation in ASD characteristics or features/traits. In his book, Nick describes in detail how a numerous features of his ASD provided the context of vulnerability to engaging with CSAM material. Some of these features included the impaired ability to appreciate the consequences of viewing images of minors. Nick describes his thoughts when he first came across the images of minors:

> Like many people with Asperger's who have little social contact, my computer was my major link to the outside world. I relied heavily on it to gather research for my studies, to obtain information about my special interests, and as a way to connect with others. For example, I would spend hours every day on the internet finding jazz music and then I would post all my recommendations on Facebook. At the time, it seemed like a natural progression for me to go from looking at pornographic magazines to viewing the same type of material on the computer. Using the computer was certainly a more comfortable and safer way to explore my sexuality than dating, travelling to Nevada, or going to adult bookstores. As I began looking at images of adult males on the computer, I was surprised at how easy this material was to access and that it was free of charge. I soon discovered that other links to more sexually explicit websites would spontaneously pop up unbidden in my view. This process eventually led me to images of minors. I was curious. Looking at these images seemed like another way to explore my sexuality because a part of me felt as if I was the same age as the pictures I was looking at. Although I felt a sense of shame when I viewed these images, I did not do so as an adult wanting to have physical contact with them. The images I viewed did not involve violence of any kind or adults shown with children. In fact, the thought of an adult engaging in sexual activity with a minor was and is extremely repulsive to me.
>
> (Attwood, Hénault, & Dubin, 2014, pp. 98–99)

Nick also talks about how he was completely unaware of the broader context of the images he was looking at and how they were created:

> At the time, I didn't understand that downloading free images on my computer in the privacy of my residence could lead to the severe legal consequences I later experienced. I also didn't understand at the time that the children in the images had been victimized in the process of creating those images. I honestly had no idea that I was causing harm to anyone. It is very embarrassing to admit that I needed to have this information spelled out for me, as I wasn't able to make that connection on my own. After my arrest, [my psychologist] spent considerable time explaining the issue of victim awareness to me. I was horrified to learn that these minors had been mistreated and that I had not been able to see that.
>
> (Attwood, Hénault, & Dubin, 2014, p. 99)

Aral, Say and Usta (2018) describe the case of B.A., a 15-year-old girl, referred to their clinic by the judicial authorities. She had been charged with possessing CSAM on her computer and distributing them on social media. The authors assessed that B.A. met the diagnostic criteria for ASD (Asperger's Syndrome) or obsessive-compulsive disorder (OCD). B.A. had been talking with an unknown person on social media. The unknown person used a fake account and began talking and keeping the conversation on the topic of naked people. B.A. was asked to send pictures of naked people which B.A. did without any questions. When B.A started to talk about naked child photos and naked photos of famous children, B.A. said that the stranger then asked her to send naked pictures of children. She conducted searches on the internet for 'naked child pictures, visuals' and sent some of them (in a link) to the unknown person. It is clear that B.A. had no reservations with talking with an unknown person online regarding CSAM, which can be seen as a strong indication of her impaired social judgement. She also sent the unknown person some naked child photos that she had previously acquired and saved from a pornographic site. She told Aral and colleagues (2018) that for numerous years she had been carrying out internet searches and research of famous children and believed this need and curiosity was something everyone experienced. She was asked if it was legal to watch, download, and share the naked pictures she had downloaded. Because the material was freely accessible online, she believed it was legal. B.A. also believed that the photos were not taken against the will of the children. Her knowledge about sexuality was considered to be at an age-appropriate level and appropriate to her sexual physical development. She had not engaged in masturbation and there were no indications of homosexual or sexual phobias. She felt a sexual interest in men. B.A. had a history of changing circumscribed interests which her family first noticed during her fourth grade of elementary school. For instance, collecting images of famous babies on the internet, watching baby bath videos, sending her friends child photos, asking every person she met their weight and size, and researching Egyptian history and the pharaohs. She first presented at Aral's and colleagues policlinic and following assessment received a diagnosis of Asperger's Syndrome (which would now be ASD) during a follow-up session. Some of the key features associated to her ASD included:

- Circumscribed interests (e.g., images of famous babies on the internet)
- Long hours spent on the internet
- Failure to make friends

Prior to the judicial event, B.A. received a diagnosis of major depressive disorder. Some of the features of this disorder she was exhibiting included: interest loss, loss of motivation, low energy, low appetite, low mood, and an increased desire to sleep. She was subsequently prescribed 50mg sertraline following this diagnosis. She was able to answer questions adequately. However, she tended to talk around the topics. Aral and colleagues (2018) concluded that B.A. was unable to understand the judicial significance and consequence of her actions due to features relating to her diagnosis of ASD and was unable to regulate her behaviour. Because of this, Aral and colleagues argued that B.A. was not criminally responsible with respect to article 32/1 of the Turkish Penal Code. Aral and colleagues stated, based on the findings from their assessment, that B.A. had not felt any arousal or pleasure watching pornographic material and had no sexual urge or action towards minors. Her behaviour was not considered to be paedophiliac. Aral and colleagues recommend obtaining a detailed history of sexual development, the motives of actions, and social-sexual knowledge. Such information would assist the clinician in making the distinction between circumscribed behaviour associated with ASD from sexually deviant behaviours (Aral, Say, & Usta, 2018).

Polygraph testing

There has been some concern about the reliability of the polygraph with individuals with ASD (e.g., Dubin, 2021). For instance, Sugrue (2017) has argued that the use of polygraph testing on individuals with ASD would be ineffective. Individuals with ASD can be more reactive to a polygraph examination compared to neurotypical individuals. Some of the classic features of ASD include repetitive movements (hand flapping, fidgeting, etc.), particularly when in stressful situations; vulnerability to sensory overload (extreme reactivity to louds sounds, bright lights, etc); and touch aversion (individuals with ASD can experience significant and intense distraction due to different types of tactile stimulation – for example, needing to remove tags from their tops and wearing clothing which is soft, loose, and non-restrictive). There are no studies which have investigated how individuals with ASD required to undergo polygraph testing respond physiologically when strapped to a chair (forced restriction of movement) in a room which likely has fluorescent lighting (causing sensory overload) while pneumographs, galvanometers, and a blood pressure cuff are attached to their body (triggering touch aversion). Also, it is common for individuals with ASD to have a very rigid conscience. Additionally, Sugrue (2017) has emphasised that this group have a tendency to be guilt prone and are typically 'truthful almost to a fault'. Polygraphers informally use the term 'guilt grabber', which describes an individual who is innocent but fails the polygraph due to feeling guilty simply at the thought of doing something wrong. Individuals with ASD have been argued to be particularly prone to this. Sugrue (2017) has argued that the application of this tool should be avoided with individuals with ASD until there is further research validating the use of polygraphs with this particular group.

Conventional sex offender treatment and ASD

The clinical utility of sex offender treatment programmes for ASD is important to address here. The main focus of the programmes include: the offender's understanding of his offending pattern, learning about thinking errors, practicing empathic responses to the victims, and stopping deviant thoughts and fantasies. While this approach can be effective for neurotypicals, Sugrue (2017) has emphasised that this approach is not suitable for individuals with ASD. Griffiths et al. (2009) argue that individuals with ASD require specialised treatment which includes very explicit sex education with a focus on learning 'specific responses to specific situations', due to their difficulty in understanding abstract concepts. Repetition is also crucial in the treatment programmes for individuals with ASD (Klin et al., 1995). The treatment programmes for those who are convicted of CSAM could cause further harm for individuals with ASD by 'confusing them about the law, their privacy rights and what and how they are supposed to deal with certain situations that present themselves when they are using their computer in their home' (Klin et al., 1995, p. 88). Individuals with ASD would also need explicit training on the consequences of CSAM (Mesibov & Sreckovic, 2017).

Conclusion

Individuals with hfASD tend to have innate characteristics that make them vulnerable to online offending. In addition, loneliness and lifelong anxiety from always feeling different leads people to search for alternative means of comfort, most commonly online (Hudson-Allez, 2023). In therapeutic work, one may emphasise that this is not a disorder but a different way of processing information, and understanding these differences in thinking styles in the therapy room is valuable, rather than trying to (unsuccessfully) make them neurotypical. However, in the criminal justice system, there needs to be an understanding that some of these innate vulnerabilities mean that the *intent* to offend is not necessarily proven.

References

Allely, C. S. (2020) Contributory role of autism spectrum disorder symptomology to the viewing of indecent images of children (IIOC) and the experience of the criminal justice system. *Journal of Intellectual Disabilities and Offending Behaviour, 11*(3), 171–189.

Allely, C. S. (2022) *Autism Spectrum Disorder in the Criminal Justice System. A Guide to Understanding Suspects, Defendants and Offenders with Autism.* Routledge.

Allely, C. S. & Dubin, L. (2018) The contributory role of autism symptomology in child pornography offending: why there is an urgent need for empirical research in this area. *Journal of Intellectual Disabilities and Offending Behaviour, 9*(4), 129–152.

Allely, C. S., Kennedy, S., & Warren, I. (2019) A legal analysis of Australian criminal cases involving defendants with autism spectrum disorder charged with online sexual offending. *International Journal of Law and Psychiatry, 66,* 101456.

Aral, A., Say, G. N., & Usta, M. B. (2018) Distinguishing circumscribed behavior in an adolescent with Asperger syndrome from a pedophilic act: a case report. Dusunen Adam *The Journal of Psychiatry and Neurological Sciences*, 31(1), 102.

Attwood, T., Evans C., & Lesko A. (2014) Been There. Done That. Try This!: An Aspie's Guide to Life on Earth. Jessica Kingsley Publishers.

Attwood, T., Hénault, I., & Dubin, N. (eds) (2014) *Sexuality of Persons with Autism in Legal Context.* Harmonia.

Bagby, R. M., Parker, J. D., & Taylor, G. J. (1994) The twenty-item Toronto Alexithymia Scale – I. Item selection and cross-validation of the factor structure. *Journal of Psychosomatic Research, 38*(1), 23–32.

Bird, G. & Cook, R. (2013) Mixed emotions: the contribution of alexithymia to the emotional symptoms of autism. *Translational Psychiatry, 3*(7), e285–e285.

Brown-Lavoie, S. M., Viecili, M. A., & Weiss, J. (2014) Sexual knowledge and victimization in adults with autism spectrum disorders. *Journal of Autism and Developmental Disorders, 44,* 2185–2196.

Cook, R., Brewer, R., Shah, P., & Bird, G. (2013) Alexithymia, Not Autism, Predicts Poor Recognition of Emotional Facial Expressions. *Psychological Science* 24(5). doi:10.1177/0956797612463582.

Cutler, E. (2013) Autism and child pornography: a toxic combination. http://sexoffender-statistics. blogspot.com/2013/08/autism-and-child-pornography-toxic.html.

de la Cuesta, G. (2010) A selective review of offending behaviour in individuals with autism spectrum disorders. *Journal of Learning Disabilities and Offending Behaviour, 1*(2), 47–58.

Dubin, N. (2017) An autistic universe: the perspectives of an autistic registrant. In L. A. Dubin, N. (2021) *Autism Spectrum Disorder, Developmental Disabilities, and the Criminal Justice System: Breaking the Cycle.* Jessica Kingsley Publishers.

Dubin, N. & E. Horowitz (eds) *Caught in the web of the criminal justice system: Autism, developmental disabilities and sex offences* (pp. 248–274). Jessica Kingsley Publishers.

Dubin, N., Hénault, I., & Attwood, A. (2014) *The Autism Spectrum, Sexuality and the Law: What every parent and professional needs to know.* Jessica Kingsley Publishers.

Eaton, J. (2023) *Autism. Missed and Misdiagnosed, Identifying, Understanding and Supporting Diverse Autistic Identities.* Jessica Kingsley Press.

Freckelton, I. (2011) Asperger's disorder and the criminal law. *Journal of Law and Medicine, 18,* 677–691.

Freckelton, I. (2013) Forensic issues in autism spectrum disorder: learning from court decisions. *Recent Advances in Autism Spectrum Disorders*-Volume II, InTech.

Griffiths, D. & Fedoroff, J. P. (2009) Persons with intellectual disabilities who sexually offend. *Sex Offenders: Identification, Risks, Assessment, Treatment and Legal Issues,* 353–378.

Griffiths, D., Hingsburger, D., Hoath, J., & Ioannou, S. (2013) 'Counterfeit deviance' revisited. *Journal of Applied Research in Intellectual Disabilities, 26*(5), 471–480.

Hénault, I. (2014) Inappropriate Sexual Behaviors. In N. Dubin, I. Hénault, & A. Attwood, *The Autism Spectrum, Sexuality and the Law: What every parent and professional needs to know* (Chapter 3). Jessica Kingsley Publishers.

Hudson-Allez, G. (2023) *A Trauma-Informed Understanding of Online Offending. Adult Losses from Adolescent Searches.* Routledge.

Kinnaird, E., Stewart, C., & Tchanturia, K. (2019) Investigating alexithymia in autism: A systematic review and meta-analysis. *European Psychiatry, 55,* 80–89.

Klin, A., Volkmar, F. R., Sparrow, S. S., Cicchetti, D. V., & Rourke, B. P. (1995) Validity and neuropsychological characterization of Asperger syndrome: Convergence with nonverbal learning disabilities syndrome. *Journal of Child Psychology and Psychiatry, 36*(7), 1127–1140.

Kumar, S., Devendran, Y., Radhakrishna, A., Karanth, V., & Hongally, C. (2017) A case series of five individuals with asperger syndrome and sexual criminality. *Journal of Mental Health and Human Behaviour, 22*(1), 63–68.

Mahoney, M. (2009) Asperger's Syndrome and the Criminal Law: The Special Case of Child Pornography.http://www.harringtonmahoney.com/content/Publications/Asperger-sSyndromeandtheCriminalLawv26.pdf.

Mahoney, M. (2017) Introduction. In L.A. Dubin & E. Horowitz. *Caught in the Web of the Criminal Justice System: Autism, Developmental Disabilities, and Sex Offenses.* Jessica Kingsley Publishers.

Mahoney, M. J. (2021) Defending Men with Autism Accused of Online Sexual Offenses. In F. R. Volkmar, R. Loftin, A. Westphal & M. Woodbury-Smith (eds) *Handbook of Autism Spectrum Disorder and the Law* (pp. 269–306). Springer Nature Switzerland AG.

Mesibov, G. & Sreckovic, M. (2017) Child and juvenile pornography and autism spectrum disorder. In L. A. Dubin & E. Horowitz (eds) *Caught in the Web of the Criminal Justice System: Autism, Developmental Disabilities, and Sex Offenses.* Jessica Kingsley Publishers.

Pecora, L. A., Mesibov, G. B., & Stokes, M. A. (2016) Sexuality in high-functioning autism: A systematic review and meta-analysis. *Journal of Autism and Developmental Disorders, 46*, 3519–3556.

Preece, D., Becerra, R., Allan, A., Robinson, K., & Dandy, J. (2017) Establishing the theoretical components of alexithymia via factor analysis: Introduction and validation of the attention-appraisal model of alexithymia. *Personality and Individual Differences, 119*, 341–352.

Sevlever, M., Roth, M. E., & Gillis, J. M. (2013) Sexual abuse and offending in autism spectrum disorders. *Sexuality and Disability, 31*, 189–200.

Sugrue, D. P. (2017) Forensic assessment of individuals with autism spectrum charged with child pornography violations. In L. A. Dubin & E. Horowitz (eds) *Caught in the Web of the Criminal Justice System: Autism, Developmental Disabilities, and Sex Offenses.* Jessica Kingsley Publishers.

Tantam, D. (2000) Psychological disorder in adolescents and adults with Asperger syndrome. *Autism,* 4(1), 47–62.

Uljarevic, M. & Hamilton, A. (2013) Recognition of emotions in autism: a formal meta-analysis. *Journal of Autism and Developmental Disorders, 43*(7), 1517–1526.

Chapter 12

Are women who commit sexual offences mad or bad?

Glyn Hudson-Allez

Research estimates that women who sexually offend constitute about 5% of the offending population (Cortoni & Gannon, 2013), whereas the Lucy Faithfull Foundation anecdotally estimate that up to 20% of people suspected of paedophilia in the UK are women (Townsend & Syal, 2009). You may notice that there is a jump in descriptors from 'women who sexually offend' to 'suspected paedophiles' even though they are not a homogenous group; these differing descriptors in research can account for the variation in outcome. These statistical outcomes maybe a facet of how the figures are obtained. For example, Cortoni, Babchishin, and Rat (2016) conducted a met-analysis from 12 different countries, and found an incidence 2.2% when looking at offenses reported to the police, and 11.6% when analysing victim report data, and a further two percentage points higher if the woman who committed the offence was juvenile. They also noted from self-report data that 40% of men surveyed had been victimised by a woman compared to 2% of females who reported being victimised by a woman (Cortoni, Babchishin, & Rat, 2016). People who were exposed to victimisation by a woman, particularly in childhood, are more likely to experience long-term mental health issues, particularly depressive and post-traumatic stress episodes (Munroe & Shurnway, 2022), so need to be dealt with as seriously as abuse by men.

Theories of sexual offending and the profiles of sexual offenders are mostly derived from samples of men and then extrapolated to women. Men and women who sexually offend do share some commonalities, for example, histories of adverse childhood experiences (ACEs), difficulties with relationships, and substance abuse issues. In addition, women are capable of inflicting just as much harm on their victims as men (Salter, 2003). But it is now held that gender-specific models are more appropriate because they do not assume that the dynamic factors associated with women who sexually offend are the same as those which apply to men. Women's life experiences differ and their offending pathways manifest differently compared to men. There has been a tendency to overlook these differences from a policy and treatment perspective, often due to a cultural perception that 'women don't do such things' (Denov, 2001). De Motte & Mutale (2019) suggest that there

DOI: 10.4324/9781003509103-14

are three reasons for this incomprehension: women can be trusted, women do not manipulate or groom, and women are not sexually aggressive. Of course, this is a misapprehension, as *some* women, although the perceived minority, are just as capable in these areas as men.

Gannon et al. (2013) proposed a Descriptive Model of Female Sexual Offending (DMFSO). Using grounded theory research methodology (Strauss & Corbin, 1998), they suggested three main offense pathways that females tend to follow:

1. *Directed–Avoidant*: the primary characteristics of this pathway are women who tend to live in either extreme fear for their lives or because they desire close intimacy with a co-offender and want to please. This co-offender may or may not be male. They may be oblivious or passive in planning abuse that has been initiated by their co-offender, remaining passive and dependent. This pathway is therefore characterised by sexual avoidance and negative affect. The pathway does not suggest a sexual interest in children *per se*, but a specific offence to meet their own or other's needs.
2. *Explicit–Approach*: these women experience positive affect and excitement in anticipation of the offense to obtain sexual gratification, *i.e.* paedophilia. They will develop an intimacy with their victim and may plan the offense to reach specific goals, like revenge against a partner or financial reward from later blackmail or promoting prostitution. Again, this pathway might include a co-offender.
3. *Implicit–Disorganised*: this is a less common heterogeneous group of women who hold diverse goals for their offending and may offend against either adults or children. They do not show any offence planning and may have disorganised offense characteristics, for example, they may be associated with drug abuse and/or psychosis. Again, this may not mean a sexual arousal toward children, but an impulsive lack of boundaries that leads to harm.

There has been some criticism of this model, and its small sample base suggests that women are less likely than their male counterparts to be convicted for their offenses due to biased assumptions about women being the nurturers of children (Bunting, 2005) as previously mentioned, but the model does have good face validity. The pathway through which a female client leads to offending has relevance for how you would work with her therapeutically. In the early assessment stage, it is more useful for therapists to spend less time on what the offence was, although clearly you will need to know the basics, but details of the offence and risk assessments can come later in the work. The client will be acutely aware of the societal abhorrence toward woman who sexually abuse children, so she will wear her shame like a second skin. For the work to be trauma-informed the assessment toward building up a formulation (Hudson-Allez, 2023), and early therapeutic work, needs to be focused on 'what happened to you?'.

Working with a client from the directed-avoidant pathway

As mentioned, the offender characteristics for women differ from those of men. They are most likely to be a mother or in a caregiver role and are more likely than men to have a co-offender. However, it has been found that only one third of women who sexually abuse have a co-offender (Williams & Bierie, 2015). In terms of their offence, they are less likely to engage in penetration of the victim, although that may occur, and the women may also have emotional regulation issues and difficulty in coping with stress.

'Jennifer'

Jennifer was born ten weeks premature and spent those weeks in an incubator. She continued to have medical treatment through her infancy with an undeveloped bowel, and had enuresis until the age of nine. She had a brother who was four years older, who resented all the attention Jennifer received from their parents with regard to her health, always treating her as a fragile child, and he would surreptitiously bully and taunt her. When she was 12 years old, her father died suddenly of an aortic aneurism. Her mother sunk into the depths of despair and became deeply depressed thereafter. She lost her job, lost interest in finding another, lived on benefits whilst drinking and overeating, put on an enormous amount of weight, and her two teenage children were left to fend for themselves.

When Jennifer was 16, she met Ian who was four years older. She enjoyed the amount of attention he gave her, always wanting to know where she was, what she was doing, who she was with, and whether she thinking about him. If they weren't together, he would be texting her, reaffirming his love and commitment, and expecting immediate affirmations back. This was Jennifer's first sexual experience, and they would make out at every opportunity, even in her family kitchen while her mother was slumped in front of the TV in the next room. Jennifer soon became pregnant as it had not occurred to her to take precautions. Ian already lived in a rented flat, so Jennifer moved in with him. As her pregnancy progressed, however, and Jennifer became tired and less sexually innovative, Ian's sexual interest in her started to wane.

Jennifer gave birth to a daughter, with whom Ian became obsessed, always insisting that he should change her nappy when needed. Jennifer became aware that Ian was fascinated by the child's genitals. She tried raising the subject with him but he became angry and threatened that they should split up, and that he would have custody of the child as she was an unfit mother. Feeling the threat of losing him completely, Jennifer decided to buy him a present: a camera. Very soon, Ian was taking photos of his daughter's vagina and posting the images online. He soon had a customer base, and the extra money was rewarding for both of them. When Ian asked Jennifer to take photos of his erect penis next to his daughter's vagina, she reluctantly agreed, on the understanding that he would not try to penetrate her. Jennifer and Ian got the knock when one of their 'customer's' devices was examined and their IP address traced back to them.

Despite having a loving family, Jennifer's birth was traumatic, and her long stay in the Infant ICU led to her developing an insecure attachment (Hudson-Allez, 2011). As such her security repertoire became one of a people-pleaser, wanting to make people happy. No matter how hard she tried, however, she could never please her brother, who used to taunt and bully her. Jennifer internalised this as her fault, that she didn't try hard enough, adopting a victim position. Her life turned upside down when her father died. Not only did she lose her beloved father, but she lost her mother and her brother too, who had rapidly moved out as he couldn't cope with his mother's depressive grief. One can see, therefore, how hard Jennifer needed to work to keep the love of Ian, who was then her only attachment figure. In her undeveloped maternal mind, no price was too high to pay to maintain the love of the man on whom she completely relied.

This is a common scenario within this offending pathway. Many such women directly participate in an offense by securing a victim or by helping to coerce a victim into sexual activity for their partner. Some are not so direct, but are complicit in the knowledge that the offence is taking place, yet prefer not to 'rock the boat' by calling it out (Cortoni, 2018). In the above scenario, Jennifer had no sexual interest in children, and therefore cannot be considered a paedophile, although she will be commonly called as such by the media and society at large, and she will suffer deeply from her co-inhabitants during her prison sentence. Jennifer's sexual interest was entirely upon maintaining her relationship with Ian, and as such, gave in to his deviant sexual interests at the expense of their daughter.

Therapeutic work with Jennifer will need sensorimotor therapy for her early pre-verbal attachment years (Ogden & Fisher, 2014), and possibly some deep-brain reprocessing too (Schwarz et al., 2018). She will also need some trauma-focused therapy, like EMDR (Shapiro, 2018), as she still experienced flashbacks from her father's sudden death. Only when she can start processing her own victimhood will she be able to reframe victimising her daughter for the sake of maintaining a relationship with a man who was victimising them both. This would require a long period of therapeutic work allowing her to build up trust in someone, when everyone in her life had let her down. Recidivism is unlikely providing she does not move into another toxic co-dependent relationship before the therapeutic work is done. As for her daughter, the physical and neurological damage is deemed more psychologically harmful due to the lack of protection and nurturance provided by her mother (Cortoni, 2018). In this scenario, it can be anticipated that when the child becomes a teenager, she will be angrier with, and feel more let down by, her mother than her father.

Working with a client from the explicit–approach pathway

'Joan'

Joan was in her early forties, happily married with two daughters. Her parents had split up when she was three, and her mother later remarried Ben, whom Joan viewed as her father. Her relationship with her real father was minimal. Her mother already had a child, Tom, from a relationship prior to her first marriage. Tom was nine years older than Joan. He was a kind and gentle young man whom Joan adored, but he had always had mental health struggles. Tom took his own life when he was 18 and Joan was nine. The whole family were devastated. Joan was a bright child and her parents threw themselves into raising Joan and giving her the best opportunities in her private education. Joan went to Oxford and achieved a degree and a masters in physics.

Joan became a science teacher at a local secondary school, and prided herself at the achievement her students reached under her guidance. She treated her students like peers and was always willing to take time with them and help them individually if needed. One of her students, Josh, was struggling with his work and she offered to help him during the break and the occasional lunchtime. Josh was 14, but already nearly six foot tall, and filling out with his focus on sport. Josh started writing little thank you cards and leaving them on her desk. Joan felt touched. He asked her if he could see her in the school holidays as he was fearful of falling behind in his struggle with science. She agreed to allow him to come to her house, and before long they were in an unplanned sexual

> relationship. Josh's parents became suspicious as he was so distracted at home, and was becoming less interested in his rugby. His mother found a half-written love note to his teacher under his pillow and complained to the school, who informed the police.

Many offenses against male adolescents are underreported, as for some young men, being with an older woman feels to them like a rite of passage rather than being a victim of abuse (Friedman et al., 2023). It is often not until much later when they start to form more appropriate sexual relationships that the enormity of what happened to them starts to permeate into their consciousness (Denov, 2004). Joan's sexual arousal during this offending process is related to emotional arousal as well as sexual arousal, as she stated that she still enjoyed having a sexual relationship with her husband, and responded to the event with Josh as if she were having an affair. Joan's behaviour does not indicate paedophilia but does demonstrate a hebephiliac paraphilia, which will need to be part of the focus of therapy to prevent recidivism.

It is not a coincidence that Joan had been drawn to give young men extra attention, not just sexually, but emotionally, due to her loss of her brother Tom. Her grief from losing the profession that she so deeply cared about, as she will never be allowed to teach youngsters again, will impact on her earlier grief, as well as the grief of the damage to her marriage and her relationship with her daughters. Again, she has an insecure attachment from her early years (Hudson-Allez, 2011) when her parents had split up, and her behaviour with Josh has led to a repetition of this event in her own life. Good psychodynamic therapy will help her to reappraise her behaviour and to reframe it from 'a bit of sex on the side' to an abusive act which may well have vandalised Josh's sexual script. Joan may not have seen her behaviour as one of power, but due to the imbalance in the teacher/pupil relationship and her role to hold those boundaries in place, it has led to her having a criminal record for a sexual offence.

Working with a client from the implicit–disorganised pathway

'Andrea'

Andrea was brought up in the care system after she had been removed from her parents at the age of four, as her parents were both drug users and violent toward one another. She was unsuccessfully placed for adoption, and a couple of foster care placements broke down. At 16 she got a job stacking shelves at Tesco, and at the age of 18 she was moved into a bedsit for independent living. Within six months she had been sacked from her supermarket job for stealing food. She met a boyfriend, Paul, who was ten years older, and promised to look after her. He gave her weed, and then cocaine, to 'make her feel good'. She soon became dependent on the drugs, but the boyfriend withdrew supply telling her she had to work for them. Andrea took to sex working to pay her rent, and to buy cigarettes and drugs, but tended to neglect feeding herself. She became pregnant, although there was some doubt as to who the father might be. Paul wanted her to have an abortion, but she argued that she wanted to have something that was hers. Enraged, Paul beat her so badly that she was hospitalised. Paul was arrested, and a restraining order placed on him forbidding him to contact Andrea.

Miraculously, her unborn baby survived the attack, but now, for the first time in her life, Andrea was completely alone. Again, Andrea turned to sex working to top up her Universal Credit and to pay for her habit. As her pregnancy advanced, she invited men into her home rather than soliciting on the streets. After her daughter was born, she continued to see men in her home, with the child in a crib in the corner, rather than leaving her alone to solicit tricks on the streets. One day a punter saw the child in the corner and offered Andrea three times the fee if she allowed him to have some 'time' with the child. Andrea was delighted to earn a week's worth of money in one hour, and told the punter that he could. Later that day Andrea noticed blood inside the child's nappy and rushed her to A&E, who called in social services and the police due to the child's torn perineum.

Andrea had a bad start in life and, in a sense, this offence was an accident waiting to happen. Andrea was born with neonatal abstinence syndrome as her mother was still using drugs during her pregnancy. As such, Andrea showed a lower IQ, impairment of her motor skills, and deficits in her attention and alertness. It was these presenting issues that meant her adoption potential, which may have changed her life trajectory, became non-existent. She experienced an attachment rupture when she was removed from her drug-using parents; for an infant, being attached to abusive or neglectful parents is better than no parents at all (Hudson-Allez, 2011). Being brought up in the care system led to many abusive situations throughout her childhood, with constant bullying at school, and predatory men seeking sexual gratification. It is well evidenced that children reared in such disordered social environments are predisposed to mental health issues, and substance and alcohol abuse in adult life (Anda et al., 2006). Indeed, Andrea was known to have experienced six Adverse Childhood Experiences (ACEs) (Felitti et al., 1998) before the age of nine years. High ACE scores are associated with maladaptive personality characteristics, 12 times the risk of alcoholism and/or drug addiction when adult, more likely to engage in sexual activity prior to the age of 15, and having 50 or more sexual partners (Hillis et al., 2004).

One could argue that for Andrea the whole system let her down, and it was her isolation and lack of social support that was the precipitating event that led to her sexual offence. She had been left to fend for herself without ongoing support, merely because she had become an 'adult' at 18 years, even though she was socially and neurologically underdeveloped. It should have been anticipated that she would develop a strong drug habit considering her start in life and her ACEs, and it would have been better if she had been offered a long-term stay at a drug rehabilitation centre in the very early stages before she became pregnant, or as soon as she attended for pre-natal appointments. She will now need long-term drug rehabilitation, and an ongoing long-term therapist, whether male or female, who is willing to become her attachment figure while she matures into an adult woman capable of independent living.

The good lives model-comprehensive (GLM-C) approach to treatment

All therapeutic work with women who sexually offend need to be underpinned by the GLM-C approach, focusing on primary goods or goals that will increase the person's sense of well-being; their states of affairs, states of mind, personal characteristics, psychological well-being, and activities, which are all sort for their own sake (Ward & Stewart, 2003). There are ten types of primary goods: life, healthy living and functioning; knowledge; excellence at work and play; excellence in agency: autonomy and self-directedness; inner peace: freedom from emotional turmoil and stress; relationships and friendships (including intimate, romantic and family); community: happiness; spirituality, having a meaning in life; and creativity (Ward et al., 2007). The therapy, needs to focus on how the person can fulfil these goals, in a subjective reconstruction of the self (Cohler, 1982) into a more adaptive personal identity and a resilient sense of self. The aim of this, also using attachment theory (Anslo, 2022), is to provide these women with the skills, values and attitudes necessary to live a meaningful and satisfying life that does not inflict harm on their children (Ward, Mann & Gannon, 2007), building on their strengths rather than focusing on their deficits. Of course, these women will never be allowed free access to children, and will also be denied, by the system, a family life, so the therapy will also need to work through the grief of that loss too.

Recidivism

Cortoni, Hanson, and Coache (2010) conducted a meta-analysis of ten studies reviewing the follow-up of nearly 2,500 women who had been convicted of a sexual offence after more than six years, and found recidivism rates to be extremely low at less than 3%, and much lower than the male sexual offender population, although some studies included sex working as a further offence. They therefore argued that using risk assessment tools developed for men would substantially over-estimate their risk of reoffending. As a consequence, the Women's Risk and Needs Assessment (WRNA) was developed as a set of gender-specific actuarial risk assessment tools designed to properly account for women's risk factors, including their criminogenic needs, which could identify potential recidivism (van Voorhis et al., 2015). However, Cortoni, Hanson, and Coache (2010) also found that women who perpetrate sexual offenses have a higher risk for general criminal recidivism. So it is vital to identify their risk and needs for general offending as well as sexual offending. As with male offenders, risk assessments of female offenders require dedicated training, clinical practice and supervision to undertake. Having said that, Freidman et al. (2023) argued that all risk assessment questions should place the woman as 'low risk' unless she specifically says that she plans to reoffend or will reoffend again if her co-offender asks her to.

Conclusion

It is vital, as a therapist to be aware of any gender bias we may hold regarding female clients who have sexually harmed a child or vulnerable adult; they can be just as manipulative, just as aggressive and even as violent as their male counterparts. Although the three examples in this chapter do not show a paedophilic tendency, an online survey reported that 4% of women admitted an interest in having sex with children or viewing child sexual abuse material (CSAM) if they knew they would not get caught (Wurtle et al., 2014), and in another survey of female college students, 2.8% reported their sexual attraction to a child (Cortoni, 2015). However, women's sexual arousal patterns are different and less category-specific than males (Chivers, 2005) with less of a link between visual stimulus and the perception of sexual arousal. Similarly, paraphilic disorders contributing to female sexual offending is also unclear with no evidence to demonstrate causation between the two. Therapeutic work with these clients needs to focus on issues over which they perceive they have little control. Elaborating their strengths and resilience to deal with their predisposing and precipitating issues can be the key to guiding them into a better way of being.

References

Anda, R. F., Felitti , V. J., Bremner, J. D., Walker, J. D. et al. (2006) The enduring effects of abuse and related adverse experiences in childhood. A convergence of evidence from neurobiology and epidemiology. *European Archives of Psychiatry and Clinical Neuroscience*, 256(3): 174–186. Doi:10.1007/s00406-005-0624-4.

Anslo, M. (2022) *Using Attachment Theory in Probation Practice*. Academic Insights. HM Inspectorate of Probation.

Bunting, L. (2005*). Females who sexually offend against children. Responses of the child protection and criminal justice systems*. NSPCC Policy Practice Research Series. NSPCC.

Chivers, M. L. (2005) A brief review and discussion of sex differences in the specificity of sexual arousal. *Sexual and Relationship Therapy,* 20(4), 377–390.

Cohler, B. J. (1982) Personal narrative and life course. In P. B. Baltes & O. G. Brim Jnr (eds) *Life Span Development and Behaviour Vol 4* (pp. 205–241). Academic Press.

Cortoni, F. (2015) What is so special about female sexual offenders? Introduction to the special issue on female sexual offenders. Sex Abuse, *27(3): 232*–234.

Cortoni, F. (2018) *Women Who Sexually Abuse. Assessment, Treatment and Management.* Safer Society Press

Cortoni, F., Babchishin, K. M., & Rat, C. (2016) The Proportion of Sexual Offenders Who Are Female Is Higher Than Thought: A Meta-Analysis. *Criminal Justice and Behavior,* 44(2), 1 pp. 205–24118. DOI:10.1177/0093854816658923.

Cortoni, F. & Gannon, T. A. (2013) What works with female sexual offenders. In L. A. Craig, L. Dixon & T. A. Gannon (eds) *What works in offender rehabilitation: An evidence-based approach to assessment and treatment* (pp. 271–284). Wiley Blackwell. doi.org/10.1002/9781118320655.

Cortoni, F., Hanson, R. K., & Coache, M-E (2010) The Recidivism Rates of Female Sexual Offenders Are Low: A Meta-Analysis. *Sexual Abuse A Journal of Research and Treatment* 22(4), 387–401. doi:10.1177/1079063210372142.

De Motte, C. & Mutale, G. (2019) How the construction of women in discourse explains society's challenge in accepting females commit sexual offences against children. *Journal of Criminal Psychology,* 9(4), 155–165.

Denov, M. S. (2001) A culture of denial: Exploring professional perspectives on female sex offending. Canadian Journal of Criminology, 43(3), 303–329.

Denov, M. S. (2004) The long-term effects of child sexual abuse by female perpetrators: A qualitative study of male and female victims. Journal of Interpersonal Violence, 19(10), 1137–1156.

Felitti, V. J., Anda, R. F., Nordenberg, D. Williamson, D. F. et al. (1998) Relationship of childhood abuse and household dysfunction to many of the leading causes of death in adults. The Adverse Childhood Experiences (ACE) Study. *American Journal of Preventive* Medicine, 14(4), 245–258. Doi:10.1016/s0749–3797(98)00017–8.

Friedman, S. H., Sorrentino, R. M., Riordan, D., & Eagle, K. (2023) Evaluating Female Sex Offenders Without Prejudice. *Journal of the American Academy of Psychiatry and the Law,* 51(4), 466–474. https://doi.org/10.29158/JAAPL.230064-23.

Gannon, T. A. et al. (2013) Women who Sexually Offend Display Three Main Offense Styles: A Re-Examination of the Descriptive Model of Female Sexual Offending. https://kar.kent.ac.uk/34546/1/Gannon%20et%20al%20%282013%29%20OPEN.pdf

Hillis, S. D., Anda, R. F., Dube, S. R., Feletti, V. J. et al. (2004) The association between adverse childhood experiences and adolescent pregnancy, long-term psychosocial consequences, and foetal death. *Pediatrics,* 113(2), 320–327.

Hudson-Allez, G. (2011) *Infant Losses; Adult Searches. A Neural and Developmental Perspective on Psychopathology and Sexual Offending.* Karnac.

Hudson-Allez, G. (2023) *A Trauma-Informed Understanding of Online Offending. Adult Losses from Adolescent Searches.* Routledge.

Munroe, C. & Shurnway, M. (2022) Female-Perpetrated Sexual Violence: A Survey of Survivors of Female-Perpetrated Childhood Sexual Abuse and Adult Sexual Assault. *Journal of Interpersonal Violence,* 37(9–10), NP6655–NP6675. doi:10.1177/0886260520967137.

Ogden, P. & Fisher, J. (2014) *Sensorimotor Psychotherapy – Interventions for Trauma and Attachment.* Norton Series on Interpersonal Neurobiology. W.W. Norton & Co.

Salter, A. C. (2003) *Predators: Pedophiles, Rapists, and Other Sex Offenders.* Basic Books.

Schwarz, L. Corrigan, F. Hull, A., & Raju, R. (2018*) The Comprehensive Resource Model: Effective therapeutic techniques for the healing of complex trauma* (Explorations in Mental Health). Routledge.

Shapiro, F. (2018) *Eye Movement Desensitization and Reprocessing (EMDR) Therapy: Basic Principles, Protocols, and Procedures* (3rd ed.). Guilford Press.

Strauss, A. & Corbin, J. (1998*). Basics of qualitative research: Techniques and procedures for developing grounded theory* (2nd ed.). Sage.

Townsend, M. & Syal, R. (2009) Up to 64,000 women in the UK 'are child sex offenders'. *The Guardian*, 4 October. http://www.guardian.co.uk/society/2009/oct/04/uk-female-child-sex-offenders.

van Voorhis, P., Wright, E. M., Salisbury, E., & Bauman, A. (2015) *Women's Risk Factors and their Contributions to Existing Risk/Needs Assessment.* The National Institute of Corrections. https://info.nicic.gov/sites/default/files/Risk%20and%20Needs%20Assessment.pdf.

Ward, T., Mann, R. E., & Gannon, T. A. (2007) The good lives model of offender rehabilitation: Clinical implications. *Aggression and Violent Behaviour,* 12, 87–107.

Ward, T. & Stewart, C. A. (2003) Criminogenic needs and human needs: a theoretical model. *Psychological, Crime and Law*, 9, 125–143. doi:10.1080/1068316031000116247.

Williams, K. S. and Bierie, D. M. (2015) An incident-based comparison of female and male sexual offenders. *Sex Abuse*, 27(3), 235–257.

Wurtele, S. K., Simons, D. A., & Moreno, T. (2014) Sexual interest in children among an online sample of men and women: Prevalence and correlates. Sexual Abuse, 26(6), 546–568.

Chapter 13

Training qualified counsellors to work with individuals who have sexually offended or who pose a sexual risk

Andrew Smith

Introduction

Approximately 11 years ago, I was training for the Lucy Faithfull Foundation on assessing the level of risk of sex offenders. At the end of the day, the then Chair of StopSO asked if I would consider running part of the three-day Foundation Course StopSO was offering counsellors who were interested in working with clients who pose a sexual risk to children. At the time, I was working as an expert witness, undertaking sexual risk assessments. I was fearful that if I accepted this offer, my credibility would be undermined, being perceived as a naïve apologist for sex offenders. However, I had always had an investment in the therapy world, having worked in a therapeutic community and later trained as a counsellor. As an ex-probation officer, I was also invested in the forensic world and in the child protection system, through working in the family courts. It was rare for cross-fertilisation of knowledge to occur between these worlds, and I wanted to change that. I was convinced that there were many very experienced and able counsellors who were perhaps intimidated by the thought of working with sex offenders – for the reasons given below – but who, with supplementary training, could make a significant contribution to reducing the levels of sexual crime. Hence, I decided to become a trainer for StopSO, initially on the three-day Foundation course, and subsequently authoring and running the Professional Certificate in Therapeutic Practice with Sex Offenders, and the COFRA 1 to 1 programme for counselling males who pose a sexual risk. This chapter is based on my experiences of delivering this training. Some practitioners attending StopSO training courses are qualified psychotherapists. However, for utility, the generic term counsellor will be used.

Emotional demands of counselling individuals who pose a sexual risk

All counsellors who train through StopSO to work with clients who pose a risk of sexual offending are qualified counsellors in their own right, trained at least to diploma level, and many of them beyond. Although trainees have significant practice experience of working in other areas, it is a crucial part of the training to address

DOI: 10.4324/9781003509103-15

the emotional demands of working with this particular client group, especially issues related to stigma and shame. As I state in my book on counselling male sexual offenders: 'sex offending against children generates instinctive revulsion and is an area of great concern. As human beings and members of society, counsellors will be impacted by such issues' (Smith, 2017, p. 9).

A statement I repeatedly hear from counsellors on StopSO courses is that when they undertook their counselling training, other trainees said that the one client group with whom they wouldn't, or couldn't, work is individuals who have committed sex offences. Many StopSO counsellors say they have uttered similar sentiments in the past. There are reasons for this. Mary Douglas points out that 'no other social pressures are potentially so explosive as those which constrain sexual relations' (Douglas, 2002, p. 194). Instinctive disgust related to the sexual abuse of children is magnified by attention-grabbing media headlines (Parton, 2006). This is especially so within a risk-obsessed and risk-averse society (Beck, 1992) that demands protection from sex offenders even though the risk of sexual re-offending can be low (Harris & Hanson, 2004). This is particularly the case with internet offenders (Krone & Smith, 2017) who make up a large proportion of a private counsellor's caseload.

As part of the Professional Certificate in Therapeutic Practice with Sex Offenders, attendees are asked to complete a reflective log. I am privileged to mark the logs, and repeated themes emerge. One such theme is fear of vicarious stigma – the fear that the shame associated with sex offending might rub off in some way, causing reputational damage. Often distressing, catastrophising thoughts are reported, for example: 'will people think I'm an apologist for sex offenders?' 'Will I be manipulated by this particular client group?' 'Do people who commit sexual offences, especially against children, deserve to have a good life?'. A comprehensive study of the above issues is beyond the scope of this chapter, although some of them will be explored below. However, an essential part of the training is to help counsellors recognise and process these anxieties, and to put them into a wider context.

Ronson (2015) describes how public shaming occurs through the world-wide populist arena of the internet and the obliteration of identity can follow. For the client the most damning conferred identity is that of 'paedo' and counsellors fear shame by association, sometimes concealing what they do from family, friends and colleagues.

For counsellors who have significant experience of working with victims of sexual abuse, a sense of disloyalty to victims can emerge, leaving counsellors feeling, initially at least, emotionally conflicted. However, a simplistic duality between sex offenders and victims often does not survive the complexities of practice. The majority of victims of sexual abuse do not go on to sexually abuse others (Hanson & Slater, 1988), but offenders against children are more than three times more likely to have been sexually abused than general offenders (Jesperson et al., 2009). In addition to being sexually abused, many perpetrators of abuse have been exposed to an interlinked set of highly stressful, abusive life experiences, involving neglect and trauma (Bentovim et al., 2009).

Counsellors can sometimes be worried that if they empathise with the victim part of the client, they will be colluding with minimisation and blame shifting. In some cases, clients can avoid taking responsibility for their offending by overly focusing on their own victim issues. However, through training, counsellors are reassured that they can only work within the client's motivational frame of reference, lest they fall into the 'confrontation/denial trap' (Miller & Rollnick, 1991). Moreover, the client will probably not be able to engage with a rational consideration of wrongdoing until the early attachment and trauma wounds are tended by a counsellor, providing consistent emotional attunement and regulation missed out by the client in childhood (DeYoung, 2015). Hence, expressed in terms of Internal Family Systems Therapy (Schwartz, 2021), counsellors have to compassionately attend to both the victim part and the offending part of the client.

It is also important to explore with counsellors why they want to work in this area. Typical reasons given are:

- I might be able to prevent or minimise harm to further victims.
- I might be able to address victim issues in the lives of many offenders.
- It is positive to work with the most marginal members of society.
- I can create something positive from my own experience of being sexually abused or sexual abuse occurring in my family.
- I have experience and skills from working with other client groups and in other contexts which can be transferred to working with this client group.

Counsellors can also have underlying motivations – often unexamined – for undertaking this work, apart from the virtuous hopes outlined above. In order for a counsellor to work effectively with individuals posing a sexual risk, clients must sense that the counsellor is able to hear about offending issues non-judgementally, free of their own agenda. In such an emotive area as sexual abuse, transference issues are apt to abound.

The 'transferential invitation' (Bott & Howard, 2012) occurs when the counsellor is invited subconsciously by the client into the psychodrama or script which is integral to the relational problems that brought the client into counselling in the first place, and which might well be part of the client's offending pathway. If the counsellor is not aware of this 'transferential invitation', repetition of the problematic script will occur within therapy, rather than relational trauma being worked through in a corrective way (Freud, 1914). Writing specifically about working with sex offenders, Erooga (1994) also notes that if practitioners have not worked through personal experiences of abuse and disempowerment, they can project their experiences onto clients. Typical projection and transferential issues counsellors can fall prey to are:

- Feeling intrigued by the edgy, taboo nature of deviant or illegal sexuality due to sexual repression.
- The counsellor wanting to either excuse/pardon or punish the client because of their own experience of abuse.

- The counsellor getting their own needs for value or being needed met through rescuing clients – often related to family scripts.
- Advocating for, rather than counselling, marginalised people because of the counsellor's own experience of exclusion.

The Professional Certificate in Therapeutic Practice with Sex Offenders requires participant counsellors to attend an hour's Reflective Practice Group at the end of five of the ten training days. As part of gaining the qualification, attendees also have to submit a reflective practice log. In addition to fulfilling the standard for supervision to which all registered counsellors must adhere, counsellors working with this client group are encouraged to find a supervisor who has experience in working with sexual offending. The aim of the log and of specialist supervision is to encourage ongoing reflection as an essential and core part of practice (Schon, 1983).

The training invites counsellors to reflect on their actions, knitting theory with practice, to promote continuing professional learning. This reflective learning should occur both on the macro level – reflecting on overall practice outside the therapeutic hour – and the micro level – being able to reflect in the here-and-now moment in the therapy room i.e. 'What am I feeling?' 'Why am I doing this?' 'To what end?' 'Do I need to adjust my response?' In training, participants' awareness is raised toward the emotional cost and challenges of rigorous, reflective practice:

- *Feeling deskilled* in looking at what can be learned from mistakes as well as when we have done well.
- *Disruption of professional ego ideal* can occur if professional competence is perceived as 'getting it right' rather than being able to compassionately acknowledge, monitor and compensate for 'blind spots'.
- *Not another thing!* Lack of capacity to critically reflect at particular times of threat, rejection or disappointment.
- *Feeling unsafe in organisations* in which vulnerability is seen as weakness.
- *Frustration of secondary gains.* If I acknowledge that I have been making too many interpretations, this frustrates my need to play the expert.
- *Disruption of core values.* If I acknowledge that I tend to become over involved, this calls into question how I have lived my life and conducted my relationships.

Given that sexual offending is such an emotive area, the above process work is a key part of the training offered, alongside the provision of knowledge. Reflecting on why one does what one does with clients is an essential therapeutic competence that has no end point. It should be an integral part of ongoing supervision with a supervisor. When working with victims of sexual abuse, the potential for 'vicarious traumatisation' is significant (McCann & Pearlman, 1990). The same thing can be said for working with perpetrators. Hence, vicarious traumatisation is discussed in training and the importance of ongoing supervision to monitor these phenomena is emphasised.

Why and how individuals sexually offend

Counsellors considering making the transition to working with sexual offenders have uncertainties about this client group that can be clarified through training. Some are unclear about whether or not it is a case of 'once a sex offender always a sex offender'. It is explained that many sex offenders have a low recidivism rate, although abuse can be persistent before being detected, and sexual offenders are up to eight times as likely to be re-arrested for non-sexual offences (Smallbone et al., 2008), although the harm caused by sexual offending is usually greater than that caused by other crimes. However, caution should be exercised as, like most crimes with the exception of murder, the prevalence of sexual offending is significantly greater than the conviction rate. Some sex offenders are low-risk and are unlikely to reoffend, their abuse taking place only in a certain context, at a certain time. Others are high-risk and should never be allowed contact with children, although even high-risk sexual offenders might not be high-risk forever (Hanson et al., 2014). Many clients seeking counselling have no previous criminal convictions, and many others are internet offenders. For those internet offenders who have no previous criminal record or history of causing harm to others by antisocial or violent acts, the risk of them sexually reoffending is low, especially against children offline (Seto & Eke, 2005; Krone & Smith, 2017).

The training course explains that there are many reasons why people commit sexual offences, and often they have more than one motivation. The list below is not exhaustive:

- Sexual arousal.
- Power and control.
- Emotional fulfilment and closeness with a child.
- Anger/grievance.
- Risk-taking.
- Escaping from reality (internet offenders).
- Attachment and trauma damage.

In my professional experience, the minority of individuals have an exclusive preference for children below the age of puberty or for teenagers. Many seeking counselling are men whose main sexual arousal is towards fellow adults, but who have a subsidiary attraction to prepubescent children and/or postpubescent teenagers. This part of the arousal template is usually kept in check. However, if in a morally deleterious or uninhibited mental state and an opportunity to sexually offend with seeming impunity has been created or randomly occurs, sexual offending can be the result.

In my training, I suggest that the people who are at risk of sexual offending can be categorised into one of three moral states:

a. Individuals who are aroused by illegal sexual behaviour desist from such behaviour because they believe it would harm others, but are seeking counselling to assist them to lead a fulfilling and meaningful life in the light of this societal and self-imposed restriction.
b. Individuals who are aroused by illegal sexual behaviour mostly desist from such behaviour because they believe it would harm others, but are seeking counselling because they have not had the self-control to stop themselves sexually offending, or they fear that they will offend.
c. Individuals who are aroused by illegal sexual behaviour do not believe or do not care if it causes harm, but are seeking counselling because they have offended and, in some way, want to lessen the consequences for themselves.

In my experience it is rare for those in the latter category to seek counselling and it is the second category of client that makes up the majority of those who contact StopSO for a service. However, it is crucial that the counsellor tries to understand the moral position and belief system of every client, in order to effectively negotiate with the client, the content, direction and goals of the counselling.

The reality of counselling this client group is that each person has their acknowledged, and unacknowledged, reasons for seeking counselling. Some clients genuinely want to understand why they have sexually offended and to be helped not to reoffend, or to avoid offending in the first place. Others want support to cope with the crisis of being arrested, and the suicidal inclinations caused through the loss of family, friends, employment and the shame of being labelled a sex offender. The suicide rate for individuals accused of, or convicted for, child sexual abuse is particularly high (Key et al., 2021) and if counselling can help reduce this rate, related children and other family members can be protected from much distress. This aspect of child protection is another reason for counselling sex offenders. Many clients are too psychologically fragile after the shock of arrest to undertake rehabilitative work, and it is often best if such work occurs after they have been sentenced and their mental health has stabilised. Clients are also sent to counsellors by loved ones or solicitors, in order to obtain a more lenient sentence, or to convince partners and authorities that they are safe to be with children. With these particular clients it is important that any letter sent to the Court by a counsellor to explain the work that has been done should stop short of making any statement about level of risk (see Chapter 17). To do so could lead to children being put at risk of harm, or the counsellor suffering the bruising experience of having to defend in Court a risk assessment they are not qualified to make. That said, a client's motivations change over the course of the counselling and can be utilised by a skilled counsellor for the good of the client and the good of all.

Therapeutic and rehabilitative approaches

Counsellors undertaking training to work with individuals who pose a sexual risk have come through many different training routes, and have their own favoured ways of working. These include psychoanalytic, psychodynamic, Rogerian or other humanistic, eclectic, integrative approaches. The aim of the StopSO training is not to recommend a definitive way of working with this client group. I do offer training in how to deliver the COFRA 1 to 1 programme, which provides a structured but flexible way of working with men who pose a sexual risk. Other trainers for StopSO also offer bespoke training on various subjects. However, the main trajectory of much of the StopSO training is to raise participants' awareness of traditional and current treatment and therapeutic models, in order for them to make informed choices about adapting their existing counselling approach to this client group.

Trainees are made aware that prior to the mid-nineteenth century, sexual crime was seen as caused by sin (Bancroft, 1974). Subsequently, it was reframed as a mental health and psychological problem, with Freud viewing sexual offending in terms of neurosis and regression to infantile sexuality. Freud dismissed many accounts of sexual abuse as his female clients' hysterical fantasies (Calder, 1999), and Russell (1986) suggests that Freud's refutations and the Kinsey Reports (Kinsey et al., 1948; Kinsey et al., 1953) idealised accounts of sexualised permissive behaviour, contributing to the fact that sexual abuse did not emerge as a widespread social problem until the 1970s.

From a feminist perspective, sexual abuse can be seen, in part, as a patriarchal continuum of male entitlement and violence against women and children (MacLeod & Saraga, 1988). Feminist insights into the abuse of male power have a significant influence on the prison and probation treatment programmes for sex offenders, developed in the 1980s and 1990s. Mark (1992) comments that much treatment during this period involved structured, confrontational interviews, pressurising the offender to describe sexual offences in detail and in terms of various models, notably those of Wolf (1984) and Finkelhor (1984).

Before StopSO was founded in 2012, most treatment was conducted in the criminal justice system, after the individual had offended. It was very difficult for an individual to find a counsellor willing to work with them to prevent offending being committed in the first place, because of the stigma issues outlined above. The treatment offered was mainly offence-focused, using cognitive-behavioural groupwork programmes. A core component of the treatment was to break down denial and to challenge cognitive distortions, including offenders being challenged by peer group members. The purpose was to raise the offender's awareness of circumstances, feelings, thoughts and behaviour before, during and after the offending. It was hoped that this would lead to increased awareness of harm caused by offending and the grooming process, enhancing victim empathy. Offenders would then be more aware of their triggers, and be able to manage them through a relapse prevention plan.

However, the drawbacks of this offence-focused approach – the confrontational style of some group facilitators and the inflexibility of the programmes – were seen to increase resistance in offenders, undermining the therapeutic alliance. Also, for some time now, denial, associated with lack of remorse and callousness, has no longer been seen as necessarily a risk factor (Hanson & Morton-Bourgon, 2004), although many practitioners at the coalface are still reluctant to take this message from research on board. In most cases denial is now viewed as a survival strategy, motivated by shame, resulting from the unique stigma associated with sexual offending, together with demonisation and exclusion from society. Hence, denial as a shame management strategy can have a prosocial component: most sex offenders caring what others think and wanting to be reintegrated back into society.

In 2017, a report suggested that the sex offender groupwork programme (SOTP) run in prisons was seen to be largely ineffective at reducing reoffending. Those who attended the treatment programme were actually found to have a 10% greater risk of reoffending than the control group who did not attend the programme (Mews et al., 2017). It was theorised that a lack of individualised treatment, the neglect of victim and trauma issues, desensitisation through talking about sexual offending so frequently or the retraumatising/shaming effect might all contribute to the ineffectiveness of the programme.

The SOTP was replaced in the prison and probation services by the more holistic Horizon and Kaizen groupwork programmes (McCartan & Prescott, 2017), adopting the following holistic methodologies:

- Strengths-based approach.
- Neurobiological, emotional regulation approach.
- Psychoeducational approach.
- Desistance approach of establishing fulfilling relationships and occupation.

The foundation for this turn from offence-focused treatment had already been laid down by Tony Ward's Good Lives Model (Ward & Stewart, 2003; Ward et al., 2007). The model conceptualises treating sex offenders as helping them to identify what needs and desires they were trying to meet through their sexual offending ('Primary Goods'), and to assist offenders to find means ('Secondary Goods') through which to meet these needs and desires in a prosocial rather than an antisocial way.

Through this evolution of treatment, what is clear is the counterproductive effect of adopting a confrontational approach with sex offenders, and the importance of the therapeutic alliance. Communicating the core therapeutic conditions of genuineness, empathy and unconditional regard (Rogers, 1957) is still the basic, relational condition of a good therapeutic alliance, itself repeatedly shown to be the most significant factor in bringing about positive change across client groups (Hubble et al., 1999; Lambert, 1992), and specifically with sex offenders (Beech & Fordham, 1997; Mann et al., 2002; Marshall et al., 2003; Collins & Nee, 2010).

In terms of counselling sex offenders, the importance of considering an attachment, trauma and neurobiological approach (Hudson-Allez, 2011, 2023) should not be underestimated. Other approaches explained and suggested in the training include:

- The neurobiological basis of trauma (van der Kolk, 2014).
- Compassion focused therapy, including the evolutionary, biological perspective (Irons, 2019).
- Acceptance and commitment therapy (Bennet & Oliver, 2019).
- The sexual addiction and compulsivity perspective (Hall, 2018; Birchard, 2017).

To reiterate, the aim of the training is to enable counsellors to make informed decisions about the approach and intervention they are going to use with this client group.

Confidentiality and reporting

One of the primary anxieties of counsellors, not already discussed, is having to report a client if they consider that the client has abused or will abuse a child or an adult. This anxiety must be unpacked and is usually attached to a number of troubling possibilities:

- How could I cope if I discovered that a client was sexually abusing a child or an adult when I was working with them?
- Would I suffer reputational damage if it was found that I was counselling a client and was unaware that they were sexually abusing a child or an adult, or failed to see an obvious indication that they might do so?
- If I break confidentiality and report that I consider a client is at imminent risk of sexually abusing a child or an adult, will this wreck the client's life and be a trigger for them committing suicide, resulting in me being called to a coroner's inquest?
- If I break confidentiality and report that I consider a client to be at imminent risk of harming a child, an adult or themselves, will I be sued?

At the moment there is no mandatory duty for private counsellors to report suspected child abuse under UK law, unlike the reporting of terrorism, drug trafficking or dangerous driving. However, there are obvious ethical and moral pressures to do so, depending on one's point of view, and many counsellors work for an organisation where there is a mandatory obligation to report child abuse or the risk of child abuse occurring.

With regard to private counsellors breaking confidentiality to report risk, there are two opposing viewpoints. One view is expressed in the document setting out the core principles of child protection in the UK, Working together to safeguard children (Department for Education, 2015), which states that child protection is given primacy and it is everyone's responsibility to report – usually to the police or duty social worker – if they consider that a child is at serious risk of harm. The second viewpoint is exemplified by the government-supported Dunkelfeld counselling project in Germany (Beier, 2016) which offers complete confidentiality to clients, because it is considered that if complete confidentiality is not offered, sexual offenders and potential sexual offenders will remain untreated, and this will result in more children suffering abuse.

Client confidentiality is enshrined in the values of the counselling profession. Whereas the prime concern for a probation officer is public protection, and for a social worker it is child protection, the prime concern for a counsellor is the client's welfare. In reality, I have not trained or supervised any counsellor who would not report if they knew that a child was currently being sexually abused. However, counsellors tend to be at different points on the spectrum between the 'Working Together' view and the Dunkelfeld view, with regard to the relative weight placed on confidentiality and reporting risk.

In my professional experience there is rarely an easy answer to when to report and when not to report; different variables play out in each case. However, the training provides groups of counsellors with the opportunity to discuss different risk scenarios, with individual counsellors revealing to the group whether or not they would report in each instance and their reasoning. Measures to help manage risk are explored, such as agreeing safe boundaries or a Safety Plan with the client.

The training also recommends the following defensible practice principles to be applied when a counsellor decides to report or not to report.

Breaking confidentiality and reporting

- The decision was made on the basis of a written, confidentiality policy signed by the client, outlining when confidentiality can be broken.
- The client disclosed criminal behaviour, or breaking child protection agreements.
- The client began to have more intimate contact with children, similar to the ages and gender of those the client has shown a sexual interest in.
- The risk suddenly increased (this decision should not be wholly subjective, but based on well-documented risk factors associated with sex offending; as part of the training counsellors are provided with a risk check sheet).
- The counsellor discussed the decision with a supervisor before reporting.
- The counsellor discussed the decision with the client before reporting, giving the client the opportunity to report themselves (if this does not put others and self at risk).

Maintaining confidentiality and not reporting

- The client did not disclose behaviour or intention that breaches the confidentiality policy, or known child protection agreements.
- No escalation of risky behaviour has been reported.

- The counsellor was working with the client to move him towards safe behaviour.
- The counsellor discussed the decision with a supervisor before deciding not to report.

For a further discussion about reporting, please see Chapter 16.

Conclusion

Training counsellors to work with individuals who pose a sexual risk differs from training counsellors to work with other clients, because of the particular shame and stigma attached to sexual offending, and the vicarious stigma the counsellor can feel about working with this client group. These concerns and feelings need to be worked through in training, and subsequently in supervision, as do the inevitable and powerful transference dynamics which occur when working in such an emotive area. Myths about sex offenders also need to be exploded and replaced by research findings and clinical experience of how and why individuals sexually offend. There is no one best way of counselling individuals who pose a sexual risk. It is an important part of training to make counsellors critically aware of the historical and current therapeutic options, so that they can make informed decisions when adapting their preferred counselling method to this client group, whilst keeping in mind that counselling sex offenders can have worthwhile objectives, apart from rehabilitation. Confidentiality and reporting are key issues in working with individuals who pose a sexual risk. Counsellors need to be supported to explore their anxieties and personal ethics relating to these matters, and given practical guidelines in order to make balanced and defensible decisions.

References

Bancroft, J. (1974) *Deviant Sexual Behaviour: Modification and Assessment*. Oxford University Press.

Beck, U. (1992) *Risk Society: Towards a New Modernity*. Sage Publications.

Beech, A. R. & Fordham, A. S. (1997) Therapeutic climate of sexual offender treatment programs. *Sexual Abuse: A Journal of Research and Treatment*, 9(3): 219–237.

Beier, K. (2016) Proactive Strategies to Prevent Child Sexual Abuse and the Use of Child Abuse Images. The German Dunkelfeld-Project for Adults (PPD) and Juveniles (PPJ). In E. L. Jeglic & C. Calkins (eds) *Sexual violence: Evidence based policy and prevention* (pp. 249–272). Springer International Publishing/Springer Nature

Bennet, R. & Oliver, J. (2019) *Acceptance and Commitment Therapy: 100 Key Points and Techniques*. Routledge.

Bentovim, A., Cox, A., Bingley Miller, L. & Pizzey, S. (2009) *Safeguarding Children Living with Trauma and Family Violence: Evidence-Based Assessment, Analysis and Planning Interventions*. Kingsley Publishers.

Birchard, T. (2017) *Overcoming Sex Addiction: A Self-Help Guide*. Routledge.

Bott, D. & Howard, P. (2012) *The Therapeutic Encounter: A Cross-Modality Approach*. Sage.

Calder, M. (1999) *Assessing Risk in Adult Males who Sexually Abuse Children*. Russell House.

Collins, S. & Nee, C. (2010) Factors influencing the process of change in sex offender interventions: Therapists' experiences and perceptions. *Journal of Sexual Aggression*, 16(3): 311–331.

Department for Education (2015, updated 2024) Working together to safeguard children. Statutory Guidance. https://www.gov.uk/government/publications/working-together-to-safeguard-children—2.

DeYoung, P. A. (2015) *Understanding and Treating Chronic Shame: A Relational/Neurobiological Approach.* Routledge.

Douglas M. (2002) *Purity and Danger.* Routledge (first published in 1966, by Routledge and Kegan Paul).

Erooga, M. (1994) Where the professional meets the personal. In T. Morrison, M. Erooga, & R.C. Beckett (eds) *Sexual Offending Against Children: Assessment and Treatment of Male Abusers* (pp. 203–220). Routledge.

Finkelhor, D. (1984) *Child Sexual Abuse: New Theory and Research.* Free Press.

Freud, S. (1914) Remembering, repeating and working through. In *The Standard Edition of the Complete Psychological Works of Sigmund Freud, Vol XII* (1911–1913): *The Case of Schreber, Papers on Technique & Other Works* (pp. 145–156). Hogarth Press.

Hall, P. (2018) *Understanding and Treating Sex and Pornography Addiction.* Routledge.

Hanson, R. K., Andrew, J. R. H., Helmus, L. & Thornton, D. (2014) High-risk sex offenders may not be high risk forever. *Journal of Interpersonal Violence, 29*(15): 2792–2813.

Hanson, R. K. & Morton-Bourgon, K. E. (2004) Predictors of sexual recidivism: An updated meta-analysis (User report No 2004-02) Ottawa: Public Safety Canada. www.publicsafety.gc.ca/cnt/rsrcs/pblctns/2004-02-prdctrs-sxl-rcdvsm-pdtd/index-eng.aspx.

Hanson, R. K. & Slater, S. (1988) Sexual victimization in the history of sexual abusers: A review. *Annals of Sex Research,* 1: 485–499.

Harris, A. J. R. & Hanson, R. K. (2004) Sex offender recidivism: A simple question (User Report 2004-03). Ottawa: Public Safety Canada. https://www.publicsafety.gc.ca/cnt/rsrcs/pblctns/sx-ffndr-rcdvsm/sx-ffndr-rcdvsm-eng.pdf.

Hubble, M., Duncan, B. & Miller, S. (1999) *The Heart and Soul of Change: What Works in Therapy.* APA Press.

Hudson-Allez, G. (2011) *Infant Losses, Adult Searches: A Neural and Developmental Perspective on Psychotherapy and Sexual Offending* (2nd ed.). Routledge.

Hudson-Allez, G. (2023) *A Trauma-Informed Understanding of Online Offending: Adult Losses from Adolescent Searches.* Routledge.

Irons, C. (2019) *The Compassionate Mind Approach to difficult Emotions: Using Compassion Focused Therapy.* Robinson.

Jesperson, A. F., Lalumiere, M. L. & Seto, M.C. (2009) Sexual abuse history amongst adult sex offenders and non-sex offenders: A meta-analysis. *Child Abuse and Neglect,* 33: 179–192.

Key, R., Underwood, A., Farnham, F., Marzano, L. & Hawton, K. (2021) Suicidal behavior in individuals accused or convicted of child sex abuse or indecent image offences: Systemic review of prevalence and risk factors. *Suicide and Life-Threatening Behavior,* 51(4): 715–728.

Kinsey, A. C., Pomeroy, W. B. & Martin, C. E. (1948) *Sexual Behavior in the Human Male.* W.B. Saunders.

Kinsey, A. C., Pomeroy, W. B., Martin, C. E. & Gebhard, P. H. (1953) *Sexual Behavior in the Human Female.* W.B. Saunders.

Krone, T. & Smith, R. (2017) Trajectories in online child sexual exploitation offending in Australia. *Trends and Issues in Crime and Criminal Justice,* 524. https://ssrn.com/abstract=3053782.

Lambert, M. J. (1992) Psychotherapy outcome research: Implications for integrative eclectic therapists. In J. C. Norcross and M. R. Goldfried (eds) *Handbook of Psychotherapy Integration* (pp. 94–129). Basic Books.

MacLeod, M. & Saraga, E. (1988) Challenging the orthodoxy: Towards a feminist theory and practice. *Feminist Review,* 28(1): 16–55.

Mann, R. E., Ginsburg, J. I. D. & Weekes, J. R. (2002) Motivational interviewing with offenders. In M. McMurran (ed.) *Motivating Offenders to Change: A Guide to Enhancing Engagement in Therapy* (pp. 87–102). Wiley-Blackwell.

Mark, P. (1992) Training staff to work with sex offenders. *Probation Journal*, 39(1): 7–13.

Marshall, W. L., Fernandez, Y. M., Serran, G. A., Mulloy, R., Thornton, D., Mann, R. E. & Anderson, D. (2003) Process variables in the treatment of sex offenders: A review of the relevant literature. *Aggression and Violent Behavior: A Review Journal*, 8(2): 205–234.

McCann, I. L. & Pearlman, L. A. (1990) Vicarious traumatization: A framework for understanding the psychological effects of working with victims. *Journal of Traumatic Stress* 3(1): 131–149.

McCartan, K. & Prescott, D. (2017) Bring me the Horizon! (and Kaizen). An ATSA blog post discussing the new sex offender treatment programs in England and Wales. https://blog.atsa.com/2017/06/bring-me-horizon-and-kaizen.html.

Mews, A., Di Bella, L. & Purver, M. (2017) Impact Evaluation of the Prison-Based Core Sex Offender Treatment Programme. Ministry of Justice. https://assets.publishing.service.gov.uk/media/5a82a191ed915d74e3402c41/sotp-report-print.pdf.

Miller, W. R. & Rollnick, S. (1991) *Motivational Interviewing: Helping People Change*. The Guilford Press.

Parton, N. (2006) *Safeguarding Childhood: Early Intervention and Surveillance in a Late Modern Society*. Palgrave Macmillan.

Rogers, C. R. (1957) The necessary and sufficient conditions of therapeutic personality change. *Journal of Consulting Psychology*, 21: 95–103.

Ronson, J. (2015) *So You've Been Publicly Shamed*. Picador.

Russell, D. (1986) *The Secret Trauma: Incest in the Lives of Girls and Women*. Basic Books.

Schon, D. (1983) *The Reflective Practitioner: How Professionals Think in Action*. Temple-Smith.

Schwartz, R. (2021) *No Bad Parts: Healing Trauma and Restoring Wholeness with the Internal Family Systems Model*. Vermilion.

Seto, M. C. & Eke, A. W. (2005) The criminal histories and later offending of child pornography offenders. *Sexual Abuse: A Journal of Research and Treatment*, 17(2): 201–210.

Smallbone, S., Marshall, W. L. & Wortley, R. (2008) *Preventing Child Sexual Abuse: Evidence, Policy and Practice*. Willan Publishing.

Smith, A. (2017) *Counselling Male Sexual Offenders: A Strengths-Focused Approach*. Routledge.

van der Kolk, B. A. (2014) *The Body Keeps the Score: Brain, Mind and Body in the Healing of Trauma*. Viking.

Ward, T., Mann, R. E. & Gannon, T. A. (2007) The good lives model of offender rehabilitation: Clinical implications. *Aggression and Violent Behavior*, 12(1): 87–107.

Ward, T. & Stewart, C. (2003) Good lives and the rehabilitation of sex offenders. In T. Ward, R. Laws & S. M. Hudson (eds) *Sexual Deviance: Issues and Controversies* (pp. 21–44). Sage.

Wolf, S. (1984) A multifactor model of deviant sexuality. Paper presented at 3rd International Conference on Victimology, Lisbon, Portugal, November, 1984.

Section 3

Thorny Issues

Chapter 14

Supervision of therapists who offer therapy to clients who sexually offend or who are affected by a sexual offence

Sue Maxwell

Introduction

Why do clients come to StopSO for therapy, and what issues set the scene for the supervision focus?

- The aftermath of the 'knock', when the only person who may know is their partner. They may be in acute distress and may be feeling suicidal.
- When the client has been charged by the police with a sexual offence.
- When the client is worried about their sexual thinking and have taken no action but know their thoughts verge on illegality.
- When the client advised by their legal representative to seek therapy because of a sexual offence charge.
- When the client has previously committed a sexual offence, been through a court process and is subsequently left with difficult thoughts and feelings, whilst trying to work towards living life in a healthier way.
- The client's partner comes to therapy because they are devastated by their partner's actions and are shocked by what they have learnt. They may plan to separate.
- The client's partner may wish to support their partner through the legal process.
- Parents seek therapy as they are worried about the actions and behaviour of their children and are seeking help to support them.
- Lawyers often refer the client when they have concern about their client who is facing charges. This is commonly because the client is acutely distraught, neurodiverse, fearful, perhaps having panic attacks and anxiety and may be suicidal.
- Traumatic situations where the client has lost their job, is facing imprisonment, likely to lose their partner, children and home. They may also fear that imprisonment may cause their partner to lose the family home.
- Other occasional issues where people are targeted by vigilantes resulting in the client's family having to relocate elsewhere.
- Where the client has experienced early childhood sexual abuse and trauma and wishes to explore their choices about their own development and possible approach to the police as other children may be at risk.

DOI: 10.4324/9781003509103-17

Terminology used

Throughout this chapter, I will use the term 'supervisor' for the person offering supervision to a health professional, counsellor or therapist; 'therapist' for the person receiving the supervision and offering therapy to the client; and 'client' for the person receiving the therapy.

Role of the supervisor

Prior to supervision commencing, it is helpful if you can agree to meet with your therapist either face-to-face or online to explore what you can offer and clarify what the therapist is seeking. It is worthwhile being curious about their experience and ask why they want to engage with you as a supervisor. In the context of StopSO work, it is likely they are asking you to supervise because they have had a client who has crossed the legal lines of sexual behaviour, having inappropriate thoughts that may relate to children or find the issues personally distressing. The therapist might also approach you because they think you can support their development, understanding and knowledge-based given the therapy that StopSO offers clients.

Supervisory contract

At the outset it is helpful to set out a supervision contract with the therapist. Several issues can offer pointers on how to help address this. These can include experience of Good Practice Guidelines for clinical work; supervision of StopSO therapists; professional body guidelines and/or requirements; limitations of your, and their, professional indemnity insurance; clarity about training the therapist has had to work with forensic clients, and their prior training and experience of supervision.

Questions that might be considered to help clarify the contract include:

- What is important to you and the therapist for the client work they are embarking on?
- What is their work context?
- Which professional bodies are they members off?
- What are the other aspects that need to be considered? For example, are they registered with the Information Commissioner's Office?

Many elements of the contract are about the working relationship and how to manage this in a way that you both agree to. I prefer to do this face-to-face if I can, or more generally online. I use a structured draft contract that I can modify and share with a therapist. They can tell me what needs to be amended, so we can reach an agreement through that process. A most important factor to consider is: what if the supervisor and therapist get into conflict, and how that can be agreed and handled by being described in the contract? Should there be a 'reporting element' required by a training course, line manager or organisation (like the NHS) that also needs to be described and included?

One of the most difficult aspects for everyone to deal with is if the supervisor or therapist becomes unwell or experiences mental health issues during the work. For the supervisor, actions that need to be taken to ensure therapist or client is offered alternative help should be set out in the contract. As a supervisor, I offer the therapist my CV and ask them to reciprocate so we both have access to the same information. Most supervisors who have completed a Diploma or Master's Level Supervision Course will have been offered guidance on decisions about supervision management and what needs to be addressed in a contract.

It is understandably difficult to think about all the elements to be considered at the beginning of setting up a contract, because the therapist might begin to work with a different organisation, or perhaps move into private practice. So, should that happen, the contract needs to be updated and reviewed by both parties recognising that it is the supervisor's responsibility to initiate and progress this.

Focusing on the supervisor and therapist

In the first and following session, the supervisor should set the scene in the working relationship process by offering the therapist a few minutes of 'checking in' by asking to talk about themselves, and how they are feeling, as an opportunity to describe what they are currently experiencing about their life. This allows the therapist an opportunity of 'grounding' in their own reality, whilst also sharing something about yourself, but keeping that brief. The therapist will then be invited to share a therapeutic issue or concern regarding the client work. Can any supervisor say what is the most challenging issue? I suspect not!

Case study 1

The therapist brought to supervision a concern about a male client who says, when he drinks and takes drugs to excess, he has sexually acted out by looking at images of pre-pubescent boys, for which he was sentenced many years ago.

Supervision process

The therapist has been here before, but this time feels as if he colludes with the client by continuing therapy and, if the compulsive use of drug and alcohol are not addressed, sexual acting out is likely to continue. The therapist also expresses worry about the level of self-harm of the client.

The supervisor asks if the therapist has ever thought about alerting the police. The therapist is clear that his primary responsibility is to the client, and the client has never committed a 'contact' offence. The therapist will ask the client to prioritise drug and alcohol therapy as soon as possible and will pause therapy with them in meantime.

Had this been a contact offender, the outcome would have been different.

Comment: the work we do for StopSO clients is seldom talked about elsewhere, as it can have negative consequences. The therapist needs space to discuss their state of feelings because of the isolation they may experience.

Case study 2

When a therapist meets a new client with an unusual presentation, they can find it confusing.

A man was arrested for taking an image of his ten-year-old daughter's back as he massaged her back and for sharing that image in a chat room, as it was deemed to be Child Sexual Exploitation Material (CSEM). What the client brought to therapy was rage at authority figures, lawyers, court, family (child protection) social workers and police, as they required him to leave the family home and have no contact with his daughter.

Supervision process

The therapist identified with the need to protect the child and saw the client as narcissistic and lacking in compassion for the horror he had created for his family. The raw feelings the therapist experienced needed to be explored to continue working with this client. This negative transference held all the defences the client could not own; his sense of entitlement: 'they were wrong', 'he had never harmed his daughter', 'he was her main support', 'he was a good man who had been badly wronged'.

The therapist was aware of the client's desire to self-protect, deny, rationalise, minimise and project his negative feelings. Gradually the therapist began exploring their own responses. The supervisor said to the therapist that there was something unexplored and not yet known in the client's process, and this may take time for the client to feel safe enough to explore further. Meantime the therapist talked to the client about a safety plan for him personally and his online safety. He had no one to talk to and resorted to phoning the Samaritans.

Weekly online therapy sessions were agreed, as this was during the time of Covid-19 restrictions. At the end of these supervising sessions, the therapist was in a different position; the therapist thought that they provided a safe space and a secure base and acted as a container for a very distraught client who had high defences and the question of earlier trauma arose.

In supervision, by responding to the therapist's interventions or comments with curiosity can help the therapist reframe their experience of the client.

Most therapists who approach StopSO are usually experienced and are likely to be to be at a very different personal life-stage themselves. We all need to recognise that we are growing and developing along with our clients. I recommend that the supervisor and therapist are open with each other, as a foil to the world of sexual offences, where secrets, power, control, abuse, shame and isolation pervade, as these can affect feelings, thinking and actions, and their experience of humanity in the wider society.

The seven-eye model of supervision with a helpful eighth dimension

There are many different types of Supervision models, but for the purpose of this chapter, I am referring to the seven-eyed model. It is a relational model that allows a dialogue across modalities. First explored by Hawkins and Shohet (1989), the model gave validation that the supervisor can experience transferential awareness of the client and therapist's process through enhanced reflection and psychological awareness. This understanding of the supervision process is further developed by Hawkins and McMahon (2020). The supervisor attunes and attends to the therapist holistically and can then offer relevant support to the therapist's understanding of the dimensions of what they bring in to therapy.

I speak from an integrative and relational model with systemic values and respect for the widest range of approaches to each client when required. I do not expect my supervisee to be like me; I expect to enable them to approach their work with creativity, opportunity and to learn how to work with this complex sexual offending client group. But many other things come in to play and I suspect the main thing we need to account for is, when we are faced with some legal issues, that we will experience degrees of anxiety. Quite often that is what the supervisee brings. The 'seven eyes' are discussed in the following (see Figure14.1).

Focus on the clients and what and how they present

To give context to how clients present, they may have been sent by their lawyer, seen a flyer about StopSO, sent by another professional or may have experienced suicidal feelings. The client may be what I call a 'naïve client' having never had

8: Transpersonal Context

2: Interventions

1:
Client

4:
Therapist

6:
Supervisor

3: Relationship

5: Relationship

7: Wider Context

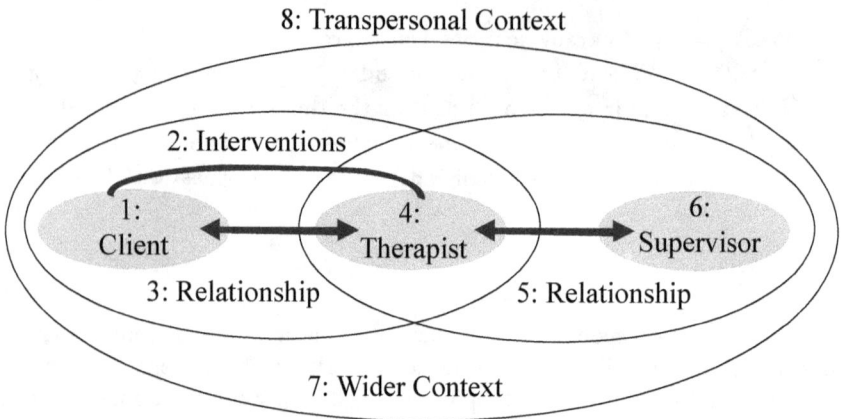

Figure 14.1 The Seven-Eyed model of supervision adapted from P. Hawkins and A. McMahon 2020

any interaction with therapeutic modality or therapy. In contact with other professionals, some clients have had mental health issues and past interventions to enable them to cope with depression and anxiety. Many clients describe early difficulties and that they have never been able to talk about what they have experienced.

Clients may see the supervisee very shortly after the client has received the 'knock' and are often in shock, with feelings of great shame, because their behaviour has been exposed by the police coming to their house and taking away all their equipment. Often that can mean taking away equipment belonging to their partner, children or anyone else residing in the same home. Clients fear that they may also lose their livelihood, partner and children. Often the partner and perhaps the children are in the house with the person who is being investigated and receives the knock. But once the police and forensic investigators triage the situation in the home to decide what action to take, the alleged offender will usually be taken to the police station and charged, potentially to appear in court the next day. At this point, the partner who is at home is kept in ignorance of the situation, knowing nothing about what has happened at the police station, and this creates even more anxiety about what actions will follow.

For the therapist seeing a client in such a 'state' it is often extremely worrying and the primary need is to assess their mental state and potential risks. So, it is critical to be able to ask about suicidal ideation once there is some idea of what the client thinks their experience has been about.

It helps for the supervisor to ask the therapist about *their* feelings when seeing the client such as:

- Do they feel confident?
- Do they feel fearful?
- Do they feel the client's detachment?
- Is experiencing this level of transference early in the therapy process helpful?

In the discussion with the supervisor, the therapist can then focus on their experiences with the client and realise that it can be overwhelming to the see the distress that the client experiences. Working during a 50-minute session can be complex if the client is neurodiverse (see Chapter 11), to ensure they are in a good enough place to leave at the end of the session.

Ultimately, that first supervision session is as much like the beginning of building a relationship with a client, as the supervisor is building a relationship with the therapist. Such a parallel process can become evident quite quickly, where many questions and curiosities can remain unanswered and unexplored. Consequently, the supervision priorities might address:

- Having a sense of the therapist's issues; can they make connection with the client?
- What did the therapist bring to supervision?
- Exploring the therapist's issues and evaluating what they addressed with the client.
- Ensure the therapist ends the session where the client is well enough to leave their room or end their online call.
- Some safety planning with the client maybe necessary in the first days of working with them.

It is helpful if some time can be taken to review that first supervision session and get feedback from the supervisee about how this session was for them. However, my personal experience is that time can be taken up with questions and seeking information about legal process, court process, mental health and safeguards such as whether a GP referral is required.

Supervising these early sessions can require the supervisor to hold the therapist in mind and provide a secure base so that they feel they have clear boundaries about the following stages of client work. There may be other issues about the context of the supervision and there may be other requirements that may have to be addressed in the future. Supervision is a marathon, not a sprint.

At the beginning of therapy, it is important to recall that clients may be very guarded about the online behaviour they are engaged in. It may well be very shaming until the therapeutic relationship is more stable, with the therapist limiting client disclosure about the specifics of what has happened. This can result in a parallel process where the therapist finds it difficult to make sense of their own feelings. The supervisor may then promote an experience, an image or metaphor that can be shared with therapist.

As a therapist, there is no formal method of risk assessment unless they have completed a specialist training course. However, therapists and supervisors are used to assessing people's risk to themselves and to others when face-to-face and/ or online. I do think that there is a responsibility to be clear with the supervisee, so they can be clear with the client that, whatever the behaviour that caused them to come to the notice of the police, they should think about stopping that behaviour.

The therapist can then help the client explore and identify the triggers that facilitated sexually acting out and develop strategies that support a safer response. But regrettably that is seldom done after the first session, so a safety plan is best implemented as soon as possible.

Focusing on the supervisee's strategies and interventions

Several questions might be raised at the outset, including:

- How will the supervisee start to assess the client accused of sexual offending?
- What method does the therapist's core therapeutic modality suggest?
- What is needed is being curious and asking specific questions, such as, tell me about what the charges are and what are your bail conditions?
- Does the therapist have an establish way of working with this client group or are they developing this?

Often the early phase of work is looking at immediate issues. What does the therapist need to do? An important element is the development of a therapeutic relationship with the client along with some idea of the boundaries that need to be in place, the support that is required and whether external organisations need to be involved (see Chapter 16 on disclosure).

Early supervision will often need to accept any anxiety that is expressed by the therapist regarding supervision, and any worry and concern for their client. Managing the client's need to devolve responsibility on to others may also be prevalent. It can be difficult for the supervisee to feel confident that they have a full picture of their client, with the primary objective of managing the client's negative feelings, possible depression and anxiety to enable them to process what has happened.

I recommend that the supervisee uses an external method of assessment, such as CORE 10 (Barkham et al., 2013), or whatever they have been trained to use, to help the client feel contained, so the supervisee can process what strategies they could adopt. Should the client have had contact with the police, a lawyer or a court, and has never had any previous contact with such a group, this can increase their perception of risk, fear, shame and humiliation. In some situations, the supervisee may have considerable difficulty connecting with a client who is acutely ambivalent about sharing any information. Within supervision, the client process is better if the pace of the sessions is well managed, commensurate the level of client distress.

Probably the most significant issue for therapists is allowing clients to discuss the circumstances in which they find themselves, and this may take several sessions. Supervision can frequently be complicated, as the therapist may want to recount every statement the client has made. But real supervision is about the process between client-therapist, then therapist-supervisor. What are the significant issues and what are the concerns that the therapist has, not necessarily the story being told?

Depending upon the therapeutic modality, I address the whole experience the therapist has: their physical feelings, their sense of the client and their sense of themselves. During that time and being alert to what is projected onto me as supervisor, my experience aims to enable some support and experiential learning and a better feeling of work-related competence. The supervisor may also notice something that has not been addressed by the therapist; perhaps a theory that may help them, that can be offered as an option as to how they may progress with the client.

Focusing on client-therapist relationship

StopSO therapists are highly responsible towards their clients and are aware how vulnerable they can be. Frequently a client will not want to approach their GP for help, and it can take some time to support them to do so. Therapists feel a responsibility to the client and help ensure that their psychological well-being and mental health are tended to. They also must keep in mind their responsibility to the public to prevent further sexual crime by ensuring their client does not act out again. But, realistically, how possible is this?

In supervision such dilemmas repeatedly arise, and it is important to take them seriously. The therapist's development is crucial to creating a safe supervision space, yet have clear, good boundaries so the therapist can model this with the client. There is a need to recognise the process of transference that can emerge between the client and therapist, and therapist and supervisor, as this can inform the therapeutic journey for the client.

I am reminded of a therapist, who even after 18 months of supervision with me, was still apprehensive of meeting me and had described their previous supervision as terrible! I believed that this therapist needed more personal therapy before returning to seeing clients. They were not safe to work with a client whose sexual behaviours had become illegal when he acted out sexually online. The therapist in this situation was unable assert their authority to help the client make change.

The therapist might indicate their client is nice; strange; scary; very demanding; absent; overwhelming; distraught; distressed; manipulative; agitated; threatening; normal; any of those descriptors will need to be explored in supervision. Those experiences can appear judgemental but addressing the therapist's view is crucial to enable their development in supervision.

Case study 3

The therapist may feel they are being seen by the client in a way that does not make sense to them:

The client, a 50-year-old man, asks the therapist 'will I go to prison?' The therapist wants to reassure him and brushes this over, changing the subject! The following is a snapshot of the subsequent supervision session that addressed the situation:

Therapist: *What should I have said?*
Supervisor: *What could you have said?*

Therapist:	*I wanted to reassure him it will be alright, and that he won't go to prison.*
Supervisor:	*What do you think this tells you about your client?*
Therapist:	*It's not about the client. I think it's me. He reminds me of my father, and I would not want for my father to be in the situation he's in. He's not a bad man.*
Supervisor:	*So, if we take that as you saw him, as if he was like your father rather than your client, what would it be like if you talked to the client as an adult. What might you say?*
Therapist:	*I could say that I can't tell you that you won't go to prison. In my experience, if you embark on making the changes you say you want to make, this will be positive at the point of pre-sentencing reports.*
Supervisor:	*Do you think you will be able to do this with the client? Something else comes to mind. What does this mean for the client's relationships with his parents?*

The therapist was able to do this with the client. It became clear to the therapist that the client had been an adapted 'good child', to the extent that, as a six-year-old, he was sexually exploited and touched by two strangers. He was so ashamed and fearful of straying into an area where he was not allowed to go, he never told his parents what had happened. He adapted even more and avoided normal sexual development for a long time. Forty-four years later he is developing his whole intimate relational experience and is now learning to accept his authority.

Focusing on the therapist (supervisee)

In a supervisory relationship there is an element of agreement about how we work. Sometimes, it seems more expert and novice. It can also be a more developed therapeutic process of equals, working together to enable a better understanding of clients and their processes. Being aware of the therapist's experience is important: how many clients they have, either who have sexually offended, or who have intrusive sexual thoughts, that are disturbing to them. Or, if the client has previously been imprisoned and is returning to do more work, to move their life on.

Supervisors needs to be attuned to the therapist's level of work and be aware of their psychological well-being. They need to encourage therapists to be good at their own self-care, and to look after themselves when dealing with traumatic incidents in the therapy space. A compassionate approach to the therapeutic work can enable the therapist to continue. Having experienced several supervisees who have required time-out due to personal issues, this may be something that has to be attended to more widely.

Transference and counter-transference issues are likely to arise when you're working with a wide range of clients who have committed sexual offences, which may at some point juxtapose with events that occur in your own life. In this situation, it is critically important that supervision is available when needed.

Therapists may also find different aspects of the criminal justice process affect some clients more than others. Learning to be clear with clients about what is known, and what is unknown, in this process helps the therapist makes sense of the clients' vulnerability, and, importantly, their own: exercising authority, to be able to say to therapists that it is unlikely they will know before their client knows. It must never be assumed to know the outcome of any court before it delivers its judgment.

Supervision must prepare a therapist for the unknown and the fear, ambivalence and unpredictability of time frames that this can generate, producing anxiety in both the therapist and the client. Such external influences can inevitably affect the therapeutic process.

For the therapist, there may be gaps in their work. The client may be advised by their lawyer to go join a group, such as those run by the Lucy Faithful Foundation. Here the client may then choose to stop individual therapy whist attending the group course, so the therapist needs to address what this means for the client and themselves.

Focusing on the supervisory relationship

The supervision working alliance enables a shared approach to supporting the therapist's development. This may be knowledge-based, require further therapy or working within the transference in supervisory sessions. In supervision, it is important to oversee the number of clients the therapist is seeing who are facing charges and/or in breach of legal issues and/or have high levels of trauma. Realistically, this is challenging work and can trigger unconscious distress and threat in both the therapist and the supervisor.

Most clients may not have a referral letter, so the therapist must have a honed assessment process which the supervisor can support the development process that works for the therapist. But, because of the darker side of this work, it is also important for the therapist to maintain a healthy lifestyle.

The supervisor focusing on their own experience

The supervisor sessions need to focus on, and be able to encourage, the widest dimensions of opportunity for therapists to engage to enable both to be creative. The need is to listen and be attuned to the therapist, whilst thinking about the meaning of their thoughts and feelings. When a supervisor becomes aware of a therapists' positive transference towards a client, and unconditionally believes the client, this becomes a complex matter if the client is being disbelieved by police and/or the court. It is tempting for the therapist to become an advocate; to be seen to act on behalf of the client. The supervisor needs to explore the unconscious process that has emerged in the context of the process, and of the therapists' need to rescue their client, with a need to recalibrate the therapeutic process becoming essential.

I am very anxious supervising other therapists – psychosexual therapists or relationship therapists – who have a new client who is charged with a sexual offence. I become very directive by exploring the therapist's level of competence and the organisational issues that may ensue. The therapist may have had no training to do this work; I usually recommend they refer on to StopSO. This avoids the angst I feel about supervising a therapist who is in unconscious incompetence, a precarious ethical place and breaching most professional body guidelines and would not be supported by most professional indemnity insurers.

Focusing on the wider context in which work happens

The wider context work can occur with some intrusions by the police, courts, family courts, criminal justice system and extreme distress. The involved family are often shocked and isolated, experiencing lack of power, shame, fear and disbelief. Often child protection is evoked, resulting in the male partner being required to leave the home (see Chapter 4). At the start of this process a great deal of the distress for everyone involved emerges.

Other therapeutic work can occur where an individual, who may be in a relationship and have children, comes to therapy with some terrifying personal feelings about their behaviour and thoughts, never disclosed to anyone. This may result from early sexual trauma or childhood sexual abuse they experienced. Usually, the reason for presenting is that they are fearful their thoughts may direct them to take actions that are illegal, such as touching a child. In such a situation, supervisor and therapist find themselves not knowing the extent of risk. There may be no police involvement at this stage, so the question for therapist and supervisor is whether any action is required (again, see Chapter 16 for help with the decision-making process), or, more importantly, how to get more clarity about what is presented. This is not something that any therapist would want to do on their own and they should always talk to their supervisor, take advice from their professional body and ensure that their indemnity insurance is adequate. Breaching confidentiality can present therapists with many dilemmas and any action should only be undertaken when all relevant avenues have been explored.

For supervisors and therapists, it is important to keep up to date with their Continuous Professional Development (CPD), especially on legal issues, advice and developments in Artificial Intelligence (AI), fast-moving Virtual Reality (VR) technologies and their significant impact on the law.

Being aware of psychological models of distressed trauma, working with people who have experienced early childhood sexual abuse, attachment disorder and neurodiversity is also relevant. In an integrative, systemic, humanistic and relational mode, the developmental process of supervision supports growth and change in the client, therapist and supervisor. The supervisor needs to be cognisant of the therapist and their own development. The therapist (supervisee) may be highly competent offering psychosexual therapy, relationship therapy and/or therapy with client with sexual compulsivity and/or trauma, but may become anxious and un-confident offering therapy to client who has committed a sexual offence. In re-viewing the developmental approach, Hawkins & McMahon (2020) discuss the integrative development of the therapist and the supervisor, which Stoltenberg and McNeill (2010) first identified, that both practitioners develop through four levels from novice to master's level. StopSO therapists and supervisors need to function at master's level as they work together to support the client to learn, develop and understand why their thinking, feelings and behaviour led to the actions that led to the sexual offence.

StopSO therapists use the therapeutic relationship to help the client make ap-propriate changes and to engage with all the ramifications that the legal process, police, courts probation and criminal justice social work, to identify a pathway to better well-being and a prosocial life. The therapist needs to enhance their profes-sional understanding and knowledge of the law, sexual offences, and report writing (see Chapter 17), usually for the defence team. The supervisor, at master's level, works more collegiately with the therapist to develop the skill to maintain their therapeutic process. Supervisor and therapist are hopeful that they can offer cli-ent the choice to make the change, when client may feel no hope The client work can be long-term. This level of compassion can at times end in fatigue. Support-ing all StopSO practitioners, with CPD training and timeout, is recommended to retain staff.

The transpersonal perspective

Considering a transpersonal perspective allows the supervisor to explore with the therapist the opportunities that crisis can evoke, with the possibility of growth emerging from that. Occasionally, when therapists experience a degree of despair when their client seems unable to move forward and change, there is a need to look behind the difficulties. Finding creative and meaningful ways to understand what opportunities may lie ahead can be challenging. Reminding therapists that their clients have lived a whole life, and their offending is a small part of that, helps to place matters in context where they can support clients to move from their recent actions to a point where they can see and achieve a positive future. Recalling and rephrasing what Eric Morecambe informed Andre Previn: 'I'm playing all the right notes but not necessarily in the right order', supervisors work with the seven-eyed model and strive, with therapists, to put this in place for the client.

Conclusion

In summary, the supervision process is a co-construct between supervisor and ther-apist with the intention of offering the best possible therapy for the client, at what-ever position they are at in their professional development. StopSO practitioners offer a unique service to clients and the public, the work is often unseen, under resourced and underfunded.

StopSO says:

We believe prevention is better than cure, so StopSO provides specialist therapy across the UK to sex offenders and those who have yet to act on their 'troubling thoughts'.

We also work with families, helping them come to terms with being related to a sex offender.

We also work with Survivors of offending, offering therapy and ongoing support.

(https://stopso.org.uk/).

References and further reading

Allely, C. S. (2022) *Autism Spectrum Disorder in the Criminal Justice System: A Guide to Understanding Suspects, Defendants and Offenders with Autism*. Routledge.

Attwood T., Hénault I. & Dubin N. (2014) *The Autism Spectrum, Sexuality and the Law. What every parent and professional needs to know*. Jessica Kingsley.

Barkham, M., Bewick, B., Mullin, T., Gilbody, S., Connell, J., Cahill, J., . . . & Evans, C. (2013) The CORE-10: A short measure of psychological distress for routine use in the psychological therapies. *Counselling and Psychotherapy Research*, 13(1), 3–13.

Hawkins P. & Shohet R. (1989) *Supervision in the Helping Professions*. Open University Press.

Hawkins, P. & Shohet, R. (2012) *Supervision in the Helping Professions*. 4th ed. Open University Press McGraw-Hill.

Hawkins, P. & McMahon, A. (2020) *Supervision in the Helping and Professions*. 5th ed. Open University Press McGraw-Hill.

Hudson-Allez, G. (2024). *A Trauma-Informed Understanding of Online Offending: Adult Losses from Adolescent Searches*. Routledge.

Hughes, L. & Pengelly P. (1996) *Staff Supervision in a Turbulent Environment: Managing Process and Task in Front-line Services*. Jessica Kingsley.

Piche, L. & Schweighofer, A. (2023) *Working with Offenders who View Online Sexual Exploitation Images*. Routledge.

Smith, A. (2018) *Counselling Male Sexual Offenders. A Strengths-Focused Approach*. Routledge.

Smith, A. (2022) *Counselling Partners and Relatives of the Individuals who have Sexually Offended. A Strength-Focused Eclectic Approach*. Cadoc Press (printed in GB by Amazon).

Stoltenberg, C. D. & McNeil, B. W. (2010) *IDM Supervision an Integrative Developmental Model for Supervision of Counsellors and Therapists*. 3rd ed. Routledge.

Chapter 15

The therapist's approach to risk and safeguarding

Dana Braithwaite

Introduction

Risk is dynamic and multi-faceted. The risk that an individual presents needs to be assessed alongside the vulnerability of any potential victim, the potential abuser and the quality of the protection that exists in the child's environment – the so-called triangle of risk (Seto & Eke, 2005). All these factors are dynamic, can change over time and can influence each other.

Webb, Craissatti & Keen (2007) studied 190 subjects of whom 73 (38%) were internet sex offenders and 117 (62%) were child molesters (contact offenders). No internet offenders were convicted of a contact offence over an average of 18 months follow up. Webb and colleagues also studied the level of failure of supervision (breach, recall) and found that the rate was significantly higher for child molesters at 17% but 0% for internet offenders. However, these studies are not current, and the picture changes quickly. Risk is now much higher due to the changing nature of accessibility to child sexual abuse material (CSAM) and therefore it increases due to a younger audience via social media. Cultural 'norms' are changing as children exchange images of themselves with sexting, creating new harms to their mental wellbeing and sense of self, resulting in complex safeguarding challenges. We cannot realistically make an internet world that is child proof, but we can make the child more resilient and savvier in this world of fast-moving technology. Social media companies could do more to safeguard and protect our most vulnerable and impressionable children. We need faster changes in law. The new Online Safety Act 2023 took years in the making, and it goes some way to help, but may be unable to robustly address advancing technologies – artificial intelligence and virtual reality – described as a fast track to a contact offence.

Dynamic risk factors

Many individuals pursuing legal or illegal sexual content online may not be paedophilic and are at low risk of committing a contact offence, if they have no previous offending or anti-social history (Seto & Eke, 2005). However, risk assessment is complex, especially for the therapist. I have formulated a therapist guide to

DOI: 10.4324/9781003509103-18

assessing risk in the client session. There is no literature to support my categories of offenders: it is clinical observation only, but it may be helpful in exploring risk and safeguarding to consider these categories of offenders or potential offenders as part of therapeutic work (see Figure 15.1). It can be considered as a broad outline tool with plenty of space for nuance. I will discuss the various circles throughout this chapter.

To add a further layer, 'spider webs' can fine tune the circles; this could include sexuality, paedophilia or a minor attracted person (MAP), sexual fantasy and masturbation, the fantasist, a vulnerable adult with learning disabilities, criminal history, attachment issues, dysfunctional family background, sexual abuse, restrictive upbringing, early sexualisation, poor sex education, lack of adult relationships, anger, violence, drugs and alcohol, IT knowledge, secrecy versus privacy, pornography use, cognitive distortions and beliefs and more that may pre-dispose an individual to this type of crime and increase the risk of offending.

As the work with the client deepens, the more circles in Figure 15.1 overlap, the higher the potential risk may be. It could be considered as a helicopter view of the client, to be discussed with the client and in supervision. If the client occupies for example 'reckless foolish' and no other circles are applicable, that number would be 'one' and represent a much lower risk than, say, someone who occupies several circles, and so the risk increases.

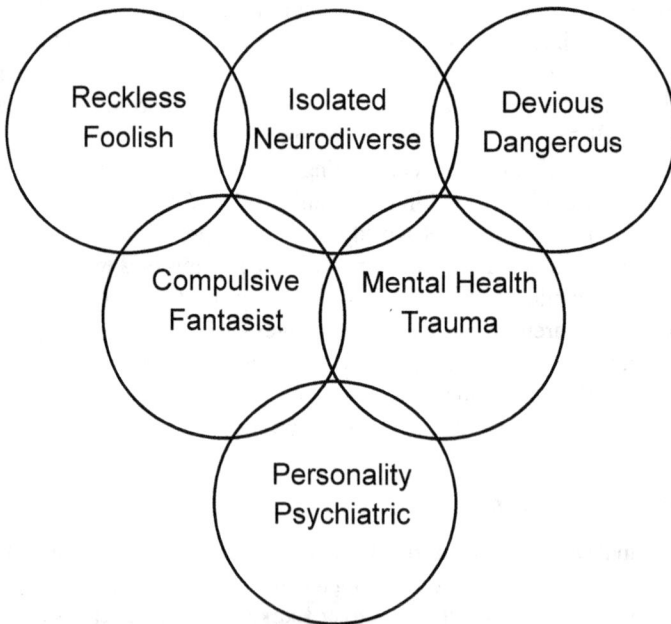

Figure 15.1 The overlapping circles of offending

The circles could be presented with the client to view and take charge of their own risk monitoring helping to address denial, minimisation and justification. It is especially useful if a dynamic has changed, *e.g.* the client has taken up different chat forums, or has been using fantasy with potential for 'rehearsing' with masturbation. One also needs to be mindful of the clients increase in stress or any change of habits, so the risk could change rapidly from high to extremely high.

Reckless foolish

This group stumbles into internet viewing child sexual abuse material (CSAM) for an isolated incident. They often bitterly regret their actions and the price they are now paying with their families. They are adamant they would never touch a child, but they were careless in their pornography access. Distracted by other events, or watched with the fascination of a car crash, not seeing this category of thrill as offending, they profess no sexual interest in children. This could be denial, or a possible early encounter to an otherwise escalating viewing of such material.

'David'

David, 40 years old, is a successful professional travelling the globe with a lovely wife and two young children, after years of IVF and miscarriages. They have a good relationship and also with the extended family. He has no criminal background, alcohol or drug use, no mental health issues, no other circles (Figure 15.1). He had a close family upbringing with some trauma involving authority. Whilst in his hotel room, he indulged in an unusual pornography interest involving women of all ages. He sought validation and attention from admiring comments on his penis. Escalation occurred in his kitchen at home whilst on a work online call. He was not paying attention to the content and committed an underage communication offence with a police officer. He missed the stated age of the child to be 14 and continued conversing until he realised the mistake and ended the encounter. The ensuing investigation found no other history or searches. He felt frustration and anger with authority and the system, aggravated by the social services investigation. David lived with his parents whilst his wife was pregnant and gave birth, and was not allowed to change the baby's nappy. David was remorseful and distressed, especially as his wife's job was threatened by the investigation. His wife was assessed for her ability to protect the children because she stood by him. She was a protector influence, and the children came first, but there was fallout and distress within the extended families. David lost his job. He was missing his children, and his passport was compromised. David received seven years on the sexual offender's register (SOR) and sexual harm prevention order (SHPO) restrictions. He undertook 50 hours rehabilitative activity requirement (RAR) and 100 hours of community service unpaid work. There were difficulties finding other work. A forensic psychologist assessment report was requested through social services and David was assessed as 'low risk' of re-offending and contact offences. The impact and distress affected his wife who carried a burden of shame and loss; however, the couple are working well together and separately in therapy. There is no further pornography use reported. He has a new job and an enlightened employer.

David now understands his offending behaviour, reflecting that the changes in his life have given him a positive aspect and maturity, with greater respect for his wife and strengthening appreciation of his life and opportunities, with two happy and well cared for children.

Isolated neurodivergent

This group includes neurodivergent presentations (see Chapter 11), learning difficulties and individuals experiencing social phobia. They often live in a fantasy world and go online to escape realities of life and others. Some present as loner types.

'Ryan'

Ryan is 31 years old and was a talented teacher. The oldest child of four, he was raised in a close and loving family. Ryan is extremely bright and well read; he had no issues at school academically but suffered from bullying and did not fit in with his peers. Geeky and awkward, he kept himself to himself. At university, he attempted a sexual encounter and was physically sick. He excelled as a Scout leader and he loved his job teaching, he spoke to staff on a professional basis only. Ryan lived alone and this suited him, accessing pornography and online encounters where he felt safe and could express himself. Online, Ryan adopted a female persona and avatar, he became 'OK with himself' online and expressed sexual interest in underage boys through this story. The boys, however, were students in his school where he taught them in class. The activity was fantasy-based and chat rooms, there were no webcams or sexual contact with the boys. There was no active grooming or intention to meet up with them. The boys were unknowing of his activity, 'they enjoyed it', this enabled him to compartmentalise the teaching and rationalise no harm at the time. On arrest, Ryan moved into his parent's home, a loving and supportive family. He was high-risk of suicide, with detailed plans to end his life, making several attempts that failed; his identity and life were in crisis. He did not appreciate the harm he was causing the students. This level of distorted thinking kept him in a dangerous place; Ryan candidly recognised and admitted that he would re-offend if given an opportunity. In therapy, Ryan was recommended to take an AQ10 and AQ50 (Baron-Cohen et al., 2001) indicating neurodiversity, which was confirmed by private assessment. He stays in his room, deeply isolated, awaiting justice.

In Ryan's case study, circles (Figure 15.1) include: isolated neurodiverse, mental health trauma, compulsive fantasist with sexuality issues, MAP, compulsive masturbation, pornography and risk-taking. There are no other history concerns. Ryan will need ongoing support following charges and conviction to re-purpose his life and keep him safe and others online.

Devious dangerous

These are people who function well in society with less obvious traits in the other categories, but with the potential for overlap. They may have superficial charm and can be highly manipulative and predatory. They are secretive and have an ability to compartmentalise thoughts and behaviour. Lacking empathy, they justify their behaviour with a sense of entitlement to which their needs override those of others.

'Mike'

Mike is 50 years old, a bus driver, married and a regular churchgoer with his wife, they have adopted male and female twins, 13 years old. Both children have histories of sexual abuse, as does the wife as a child. Mike was accused of incest with his adopted daughter. The police were involved, but no further action was taken through lack of evidence. Mike privately confessed the allegation in the family, and safeguarding is in place at the church. Social services were involved; he moved out of the family home but returned when the daughter moved out. His marriage was not a sexual one. He did not use pornography and undertook little masturbation. Previously in a position of responsibility with young girls, he engaged in subtle grooming with his kind and caring nature. He had behaved inappropriately in the past, but it was not reported. His persona is 'the saviour,' seeking to be liked by everyone. The couple are wanting to get back into 'helping' roles in the church again, and this is where the risk potential is high. He admits to being attracted to young post-pubescent females, and the wife appears not to be a protector influence in seeing the risks involved (Figure 15.1).

Mike is in the devious dangerous circle (Figure 15.1), deceptive and highly manipulative to all around him. He is skilled in the art of grooming. It takes time for him to reveal all facets of his personality and it is difficult to see how further therapy at this time can help him, as he also manipulates the focus of the therapy. He is very high risk and flying under the radar.

Compulsive fantasist

Despite negative consequences, this type is compulsive and impulsive in other ways. He can be a risk taker, seeking dopamine highs and instant gratification. He believes sexual fantasy chats are OK, and cause no harm: 'there is no such thing as the thought police'. He is often pre-occupied with sex and escalation of fantasy. The therapist needs to know how much time the individual spends in online activity, showing the level of pre-occupation and escalation. This is often linked to early sexualisation through pornography addiction as discussed in Chapter 7.

'Peter'

Peter is a highly intelligent professional man and well respected in the community, charismatic and engaging. He was married with no children. He was caught downloading child sexual abuse material (CSAM) and sentenced to 12 months in prison, suspended for two years. He was placed on the sexual offender's register, (SOR) received a sexual harm

prevention order, (SHPO) and was required to undertake 50 rehabilitative activity requirement days (RAR), 150 hours community service
work, plus a Horizon course (group sex offender treatment course). He
lost his job, his home, his wife and his reputation. Peter was a compulsive masturbator, up to four times a day, in addition to regular sexual
activity with his wife. Although they watched pornography together,
Peter felt insecure. He was brought up in a wealthy family with nannies
and two brothers, one of whom was fostered. Peter was clever and
valued for his intelligence but had attachment issues. He was a perfec-
tionist and could always find his way out of trouble. He was sexualised
early by an introduction to pornography. He found talking to girls difficult, but then met his wife at university, his only sexual partner. Peter
has struggled to manage sexual fantasy, objectification and masturbation, escalating risks and masturbating in the car park at work. He goes
to a support group, yet still binges on pornography occasionally after
months of sobriety. He is attracted to young pre- and post-pubescent
girls, struggling to manage his gaze in public with later fantasy. He
knows this could lead to him crossing the line and continues to take
risks by finding ways around software blocking, and deleting material he
hopes will be undetected, leading to him breaking his sexual harm prevention order (SHPO) and a further court appearance. Peter is lonely
and struggling to find a new identity. He realised he could re-offend if
he accessed pornography to fantasise. He has no children in his life or
extended family; he assessed his contact offence risk as low and re-
offending risk as medium. Peter used to drink heavily and took various
drugs, but no longer does. He also liked to spend money impulsively.

Peter is in the compulsive fantasist circle (Figure 15.1) with some overlap into
devious, as he likes to 'get away with it'. There is no reported mental health history
or personality diagnosis. The 'spider webs' include risk-taking behaviour, breaking rules, impulsivity, alcohol and drug intake (which is now reduced), a sense of
entitlement and perfectionism with insecure attachments. In therapy, we acknowledged his struggles and celebrated his achievements and efforts. We listen out for
the sudden unimportant decisions (SUD), a self-talk of innocent reasoning, *e.g.* to
buy a present online, which takes him down the rabbit hole into dangerous fantasy.

Trauma and mental health (damaged souls)

Trauma histories, adverse childhood experiences (ACE), dysfunctional back-
grounds and attachment issues can all lead to enduring mental health difficulties.

Seeking connections and relief from emotional pain in the present and the past can also lead to distorted thinking patterns from their own history of sexual abuse and other traumas, becoming vulnerable adults.

'Ray'

Ray, 35 years old, was working in a stressful job in the NHS. He was intelligent, with deep anger issues permeating every corner of his life and was admitted voluntarily to a psychiatric hospital. He self-harms and experiences suicidal ideation and road rage. He has little tolerance towards other adults who offend him. Ray suffered mental and sexual abuse by a family member from aged four to his teens. His family were dysfunctional, with mental health issues, lack of boundaries, physical abuse and generational sexual abuse. His distorted thinking around sex is 'sex means you like me', so he sought sexual attention to receive affection. The extended family, who also have abusive histories and lack of boundaries, put their young child of five years old at risk by en-couraging the child to see Ray on her own. She has seen him naked and touched his penis. The child refers to him as her boyfriend. There is an investigation by the police, although a further rape case against him was dropped. Ray confessed to the police about his online and offline be-haviours and fully expects to serve a prison sentence. Ray has taken his own abuser to court for historical child abuse. He has lost his job due to the stress of the investigation of both crimes. He is in a relationship with a lady with her own mental health, trauma and sexual abuse issues. Ray, though insightful, has struggled to re-frame his distorted thinking styles and exhibits signs of ADHD and PTSD. Ray is on medication, and knows his mental health suffers if he accesses pornography even if he uses it to soothe his mental health stress. He therefore needs to find appropriate outlets for his anger and stress and states he is not inclined to offend again. Interestingly, Ray is now starting to experience the childlike fun he missed as a child. His risk remains high.

Ray is a 'damaged soul' in the trauma/mental health circle (Figure 15.1) but over-laps with compulsive fantasist, devious, dangerous and personality/psychiatric. His 'spider webs' are undiagnosed mental health and BPD (borderline personal-ity disorder) and emotional dysregulation. Ray's history of familial sexual abuse, maintained by poor mental health and anger, will pre-dispose an individual to this type of crime. Ray has a long history of disturbance and realises he is attracted to children, and is re-traumatising himself with his offending: 'this is what happens to children'.

Suicidal ideation

These clients often do not present with any identifiable mental health conditions until after 'the knock'. Then depression and anxiety are common; it is a high-risk time for the alleged offender to feel overwhelmed with grief, shame and loss, seeing the impact and pain on his family. As he confronts this aspect of himself, and reveals his self-loathing, he may feel that his only option is to take steps to actively commit suicide. The world of a respectable or ordinary individual in society collides with the secretive deviant side of his personality, which over many years have been kept apart. It is important early on to address the intent, method and timing of a potential suicidal decision, seek medical help quickly for anti-depressants as therapy starts to address the challenges and explore the inner world. The crisis may have revealed underlying levels of slowly diminishing mental health and lack of self-awareness. There are often reported feelings of relief that the burden of his offending is now to be addressed despite the legal consequences he must face.

Mental health

The role mental health plays is a principal factor in the question that needs to be asked 'does mental health play a significant role in carrying out this offence?' from a legal perspective. Increasingly, patients are presenting in mental health services with concerns over their thoughts and behaviours whilst under a particular stress. The NHS is ill-equipped with the skills and resources to deal with this aspect of mental health. Alcohol use is not a mitigating factor. Risk factors to consider include isolation, being unable to engage in close intimate relationships and personality disorders. Clearly, not all individuals with mental health issues go on to commit sexual offences. In the same vein, not all individuals who were sexually abused go on to commit the sexual abuse of others. It is how the presenting mental health manifestation is considered alongside other factors in assessing overall risk and safeguarding that determines how much this is an influence overall at the time of offence.

Psychoeducation helps to reduce risk and works with prevention strategies, yet some clients find restrictions hard to accept. A full history is invaluable to understanding the world this group occupies: early trauma and sexualisation, and the role of pornography and the internet which plays in the interface of connections with others. An exploration of shopping habits, time spent on the internet game-playing and discovering a list of their most common 'go to' sites, not just sexual sites, provides a backdrop to the relationship with the internet.

Further risk factor check list – the client

This is a further checklist of red flags to consider if the client exhibits risk behaviours and/or attitudes (the highest risk is in bold).

- **Has court appearances for sexual offences.**
- **Has been accused of sexual offending more than once.**
- **Has sexually offended against unrelated victim (did not know the victim 24 hours before the offence).**
- **Has committed a contact sexual offence against a pre-pubescent male.**
- Has an exclusive sexual preference for children.
- Has a pattern of meeting social, emotional and esteem needs predominantly through children rather than adults.
- Is currently abnormally sexually pre-occupied.
- Has a strong sense of sexual entitlement.
- Has a history of violence (including domestic abuse).
- Believes that children enjoy sex and are sexually seductive.
- Has a current pattern of grievance thinking.
- Has a pattern of callousness.
- Has a current pattern of lifestyle impulsiveness.
- Has a history of chaotic/shallow attachments.
- Has dropped out of group or therapy programmes.
- Has poor cognitive problem solving.
- Has current substance misuse problems.
- **Is in contact with children of the same age and sex he has shown deviant interest in.**
- **Is an intimidating presence in the home where the child at risk resides.**
- **The child's at-risk parent/s do not recognise the risk posed by the client.**

(Smith, 2018)

Safeguarding the therapist

The therapist may have been working for some time with a client as he waits for the long process of the criminal justice system to complete. You may be approached by the investigating police officer with a signed consent form to release your notes, as your client has signed a generic consent form. A polite refusal at this stage is needed as the therapeutic confidentiality is at risk: these forms are a request for access to a medical report (Hudson-Allez, 2004). The time to produce any report is after the solicitor/barrister has requested one from you for the case once the charges are known. The report is written to aid the court in their decision making and not written in defence of the client (see Chapter 17).

Review the contract regularly to cover confidentiality, disclosure and report writing, whether you choose to write one or not. The therapist's job is to work with the client in therapy, not to police him. There is a delicate balance here to assist justice. Unless you are a trained forensic psychologist/social worker, even though you know your client better than anyone else over your time working with him, you cannot assess your own client for a formal opinion or comment on risk. It is the independent assessor who explores static and dynamic risk factors without the bias of a relationship with the offender (Bridges, 2006). You are creating a space for the client to trust and work with you to explore their thoughts and processing; you are learning to challenge and listen with a third ear, as some clients are manipulative and secretive. I have found in clinical practice that helping the client to assess their own risk and trigger points and seeing how they approach this may reveal more to and about themselves, and the therapist is wise to balance static and dynamic risks informally through their own reflective processes, developing skills to see the blind-spots and cognitive distortions. Therapists do not always get the full picture either.

There are challenges if it is disclosed to you by the client (rare) that he is currently contact abusing a child. This becomes an issue around child-protection, confidentiality and disclosure, not secrecy and colluding, and should be discussed immediately in supervision (see Chapter 13). In challenging the offender to help him see his offence as maintaining criminality through the lens of being a 'consumer of a product', he can learn he has choices to make by not accessing CSAM, which is preventing further harm and helping him to see his responsibility for change. You may not see the partner (Chapter 8), but you are assessing the relationship and the partner's ability to protect any children in the household, although social services are usually involved at this stage (Chapter 4).

Checking his understanding of the circles (Figure 15.1) will help to reduce risk and re-offending behaviour **for the longer term** and help his readjustment and rehabilitation. He must do the work; the responsibility for the client's actions lies with the client, not with you, the therapist.

Working safely online

Undertaking therapeutic work with StopSO clients is not conventional sex therapy. Here are some guidelines on how to work with them safely online: sex therapists are, understandably, comfortable in talking about sex. But it might be the very prospect of having sexually explicit conversations with someone online or in a therapy room that turns a client on. They may lack the understanding of how to behave, and thus may become flirtatious, making sexual innuendo or even overtly becoming sexually aroused to tempt or alternatively shock the therapist into a response. Or you might have a client who has autistic traits (Chapter 11), or who has a trauma history of sexual abuse and has internalised it as being 'normal' to be sexualised with strangers. A clear form of contracting with the client at the outset is essential, ensuring the client is made aware of the parameters in which you will be working/practicing, and as the work progresses, finding what is acceptable and unacceptable behaviour.

A helpful question to ask ourselves is, 'is anything sexual okay in the therapy room, both in words and deed?' People who cross the line into a forensic population usually have very distorted boundaries, or a complete lack of boundaries, regarding other people around them. So, we need to think about the type of issue the client is being referred for, and to check out what triggers a client into thinking that is okay for them to cross the line. For example, a client who does not understand that when women look at him in the street and smile at him, this does not mean they want to have sex with him. In addition, such clients may have significant trauma histories and/or attachment difficulties (Hudson-Allez, 2011) and thus have never been taught what is a proper boundary to keep. There is a wealth of literature that strongly shows that most men and some women who cross the line and violate sexual boundaries with children and adults do have distorted thinking styles, so if you think you know how the client may respond in certain situations, it is fallacious.

Most of the clients we see will know that, for example, wanting to have sex with a child is wrong. But some may well believe that it is not harmful and may see children as 'sexually knowing' and 'able to cope with sexual contact with an adult', or that it is a mutually consensual love relationship. Such cases are not unusual, where the client's thinking style has become so distorted through looking at so many images of sexually abused and exploited children that they argue that the children looked happy because they were smiling, so they must have they liked it (Van-Leeson & Hudson-Allez, 2020).

Safeguarding the client

We need to safeguard the client from himself, in particular from suicidal thoughts and attempts, which is highest following the 'knock', by being mindful of suicidal risk and informing others like the GP and/or secondary mental health team, or relatives if you have the consent to do so. Within the therapy itself, it is raising his awareness and education around dynamic risk factors, his strategies to manage and not put himself at risk of re-offending, to prevent further harm to himself and others. This needs the involvement, not policing, of those around him, knowing the strategies to support, so they can protect and safeguard, thereby reducing risk so it becomes second nature to follow the strategies. This, though, can create a burden of responsibility on the partner, who themselves are a secondary victim in the crime (see Chapters 3 and 8). Internet offenders are increasingly at risk of breaching their SHPO (sexual harm prevention order) via private browsing history and automatic deleting of history through the Google 90-day auto-delete, or other providers who automatically delete history, therefore settings need checking quickly and regularly.

Future risk, working within limitations

Most of our clients do not identify themselves as paedophiles due to the vilification and fear of the media and public. Most of our clients say they would never touch a child, yet some do. We cannot predict future risk given the dynamic and multi-faceted nature of this crime. Where it is felt that a risk is high with multiple red flags, then a Forensic Risk Assessment may be needed, usually provided for the courts to help decide sentencing.

For the StopSO therapist, self-care is important; seek support, recognise your limitations and use specialist supervision well, with a StopSO supervisor and group peer support.

Summary

Whilst risk and safeguarding concern us all, it is dynamic in its form and uniquely individual. No-one knows the client as well as the skilled therapist to informally assess the level of risk at each session. Do not be afraid to consider it closely with the client by checking out their understanding and setting boundaries and goals. It takes time to build the trust and rapport to challenge the client appropriately. This is the skill and role of individual therapy to compassionately support the client to build their own coping skills and mechanisms to reduce the risk of re-offending, whether it is internet or contact offences. Specialist supervision is essential.

We adopt the Good Lives Model (Ward & Brown, 2004: Harkins et al., 2012) and work with offenders to find less harmful and legal outlets for sexual desires with a new sense of self and identity. If clients can just desist, they may do so for a while, particularly whilst the eye of the legal system is upon them and they are motivated by fear of the consequences, but what happens when they move into a period of temptation, triggers and complacency? Over the longer term, the strategies adopted must be robust and become almost unconscious in practice. If you take offending out, then there needs to be something meaningful in life to replace it, so there is a need to examine further constructive interventions to 'help and change' as opposed to just control (Bridges, 2006).

StopSO therapists provide a tailored service to work alongside the offender to protect the victims, the family and society. Trained therapists are uniquely placed to continue to assess risk and safeguarding to the best of their knowledge and abilities, challenging the offenders to question their own motivations and adjust strategies with compassion without collusion. Clients need to own their risk dynamic and what to do with it, and where to go when they are struggling. They may look to understand their behaviour, but it is their actions that count. Few professionals have the skills to explore the intimate relationships and devastating impact on the partner and their families, extended families, working lives and wider relationships as a StopSO therapist.

Society globally is faced with great ethical challenges through artificial intelligence (AI) and virtual reality (VR) pulling in younger and vulnerable potential offenders. We ignore this at our peril, as it changes everything. It even changes how we deliver therapy, happening now through 'bots'. StopSO therapists work is invaluable to offer the chance to restore mental health, wellbeing and meaningful lives through healthy real-world connections and relationships. It is challenging but satisfying work when clients grow and change, becoming aware of their own risk potential and it is not work for the faint-hearted. Our criminal justice system can only do so much, we must keep up and adapt. This is a multidisciplinary societal and cultural approach. Globally, our children have never been more at risk.

Controversially, for those who cannot adapt behaviours by themselves, there is a role for libido-reducing medication for a minority. Those offenders who are open to change, can change, but if nothing changes, nothing changes.

References

Baron-Cohen, S., Wheelwright, S., Skinner, R., Martin, J. & Clubley, E. (2001) The Autism-Spectrum Quotient (AQ): Evidence from Asperger Syndrome/High Functioning Autism, Males and Females, Scientists and Mathematicians. *Journal of Autism and Developmental Disorders,* 31(1), 5–17. https://doi.org/10.1023/A:1005653411471.

Bridges, A. (2006) An Independent Review of a Serious Further Offence Case: Anthony Rice. HM Inspectorate of Probation. https://www.justiceinspectorates.gov.uk/probation/wp-content/uploads/sites/5/2014/03/anthonyricereport-rps.pdf.

Harkins, L., Flak, V. E., Beech, A., & Woodhams, J. (2012). Evaluation of a community-based sex offender treatment program using a Good Lives Model approach. *Sexual Abuse: A Journal of Research and Treatment,* 24(6), 519–543. https://doi.org/10.1177/1079063211429469.

Hudson-Allez, G. (2004) Threats to psychotherapeutic confidentiality: Can psychotherapists in the UK really offer a confidentiality ethic to their clients? *Psychodynamic Practice,* 10(3), 317–331. https://doi.org/10.1080/14753630410001733967.

Hudson-Allez, G. (2011) *Infant Losses; Adult Searches. A Neural and Developmental Perspective on Psychopathology and Sexual Offending.* 2nd ed. Karnac.

Online Safety Act 2023 (c.50) https://www.legislation.gov.uk/ukpga/2023/50/enacted.

Seto, M. C. & Eke, A. W. (2005) The criminal histories and later offending of child pornography offenders. *Sexual Abuse: A Journal of Research and Treatment,* 17(4), 201–210. https://doi.org/10.1177/107906320501700209.

Smith, A. (2018) *Counselling Male Sexual Offenders: A Strengths-Focused Approach.* Routledge.

Van-Leeson, T. & Hudson-Allez, G. (2020) Should StopSO provide therapists with guidelines when dealing with Forensic StopSO clients online? A conversation between Dr Terri Van-Leeson and Dr Glyn Hudson-Allez. Online seminar presented on 17 November 2020.

Ward, T. & Brown, M. (2004) The Good Lives Model and conceptual issues in offender rehabilitation. *Psychology, Crime & Law, 10*(3), 243–257. https://doi.org/10.1080/1068316041000166244.

Webb, l., Craissatti, J. & Keen, S. (2007) Characteristics of child pornography offenders: a comparison with child molesters. *Sex Abuse: A Journal of Research and Treatment,* 19(4), 449–465. https://doi.org/10.1177/107906320701900408.

Chapter 16

Making disclosures of crime or serious harm

Matthew Graham

Introduction

A StopSO therapist may receive from a client a confession, or other information, that they have committed a crime, are planning or expecting to commit a crime or are otherwise engaging in harmful, risky thought or behaviour. Such a scenario will raise the question as to whether that information should or must be shared with others. This chapter does not consider the disclosure of self-harm or suicide, which is an important but separate issue, addressed in Chapters 1 and 7. This chapter seeks to go to the heart of a crucial question: 'do I have to report my own client?'. As we will see, it is rare that a therapist *must* report their own client – there is no general overarching legal duty to report a client even when they make the most serious of disclosures. However, a combination of the legal, ethical and therapeutic duties makes the reality of such a decision much more complex and nuanced.

Framework

The principles of data protection and confidentiality mean that the starting point in deciding whether or not disclosure is required is always that information obtained during the therapeutic relationship is considered private and should remain so. This principle of confidentiality is very important both legally, ethically and therapeutically. There is no generally legal duty to disclose.

However, from this starting point, there are a number of scenarios where a therapist, when handling information which is otherwise confidential, either *must* disclose or *may* disclose.

If a therapist encounters a *must* disclose situation, then they have no choice. These must disclose scenarios arise from particular legal, statutory obligations. Here, the law compels the therapist to make a disclosure whether they like it or not, irrespective of any ethical or therapeutic consequence. These scenarios are rare in typical practice, but important if and when they arise.

If a therapist encounters a *may* disclose situation then a choice arises: whether to disclose at all, and if so to whom and to what extent. In typical practice such scenarios may be quite common.

DOI: 10.4324/9781003509103-19

Therapists working with children will have further considerations, which are beyond the scope of this chapter and are discussed in Chapters 4 and 10. Therapists in 'close proximity' to a third person directly impacted by a disclosure may also have other considerations, and should seek specific support from their supervisor (see Chapter 14); for example this might include where a therapist is supporting more than one connected person, or where something arises in connection with their own family or close friend.

There are also scenarios when a client authorises or positively requests a report or the sharing of otherwise confidential material. The therapist may or may not agree, but a competent client has the right to direct the use of their otherwise confidential information howsoever they choose. Where the thinking of the therapist and client is not aligned, the therapist should usually seek further guidance from their supervisor. Difficult examples include where a disclosure might be for an improper purpose (such as with intent to harm a victim); where it would be administratively burdensome; or where there is significant debt owed. It might be thought that recent decades have seen a growing pressure on therapeutic professionals. On the one hand, the law and principles of data protection have increased requirements to keep confidential information private. On the other hand, the long overdue unmasking of institutional cover ups and a better emphasis on safeguarding training sees ever greater pressure to report.

If a therapist arrives at a stage where a disclosure is to be made, the question of to whom and the extent of the disclosure must arise. This will usually involve making a disclosure to the police via a report to 101 or online to the force most closely associated with the events in question. Sometimes it will involve a report to the local authority, usually via the children's social care team at the most relevant local council. In other instances, a report may be made directly to a multi-agency public protection group, a probation officer or other professional. Therapists may encounter disclosure decisions to another non-professional civilian, but this will be rare. Disclosures can sometimes properly be made anonymously, although a therapist should be careful to consider whether this would meet the legal or ethical duty in the case. Any disclosure should go no further than is necessary and proportionate. Bear in mind that the police in particular can always ask for more information if they need it, and even take steps to compel disclosure should it be required. Making the disclosure does not mean a therapist will be asked to provide a witness statement to police. The ethical or legal duty to disclose may be met without giving a statement. Alternatively, providing a witness statement if asked might be consistent with the legal or ethical duty that leads to the disclosure in the first place.

Circumstances in which a therapist must disclose

A detailed analysis and discussion about the following *must* disclose scenarios is beyond the scope of this chapter. These bullet points may help a therapist recognise *must* disclose situations, but further advice should be sought if they arise in practice.

- *Terrorism offences*: the Terrorism Act 2000 penalises, with the threat of imprisonment, persons who fail to disclose varying degrees of knowledge, belief or suspicion of the commission by others of terrorist offences. Therapists who may encounter issues or terrorism or radicalisation should also be familiar with the counter terrorism policing 'Prevent' programme and surrounding initiatives.
- *Female genital mutilation*: Section 5B of the Female Genital Mutilation Act 2003 contains a legal, mandatory duty to report known cases of female genital mutilation (FGM) in girls under the age of 18. The legislation requires a healthcare professional, teacher or social care worker to make a report to the police where, in the course of their professional duties, they discover FGM. Whether a particular therapist works in a regulated professional organisation for these purposes, or works independently, will be case specific. However, if the duty is not a *must* disclose scenario as they work in private practice, it might amount to a desire or wish to disclose scenario.
- *Court order or witness summons*: it is possible for a court to issue an order that a therapist make a disclosure of certain documents – such as written notes of any sort – or that the therapist attends at court with such documents to hand over. A therapist may be summonsed to court to give evidence or to be deposed as a witness. Such orders are rare but are usually very clear. Such an order must be complied with strictly and to the timescale stated in the order. Failure to comply will be a very serious matter. It should be noted that a court order is different from a police request for information. The police are perfectly entitled to make a reasonable request for information from a therapist if it is a legitimate line of enquiry. This may arise either because the therapist has worked with a victim or perpetrator (or both). A therapist may professionally and properly decline such a police request. Whether they should do so will require a balancing of other factors (see below).
- *Other statutory obligations*: there are various other scenarios in which the law requires a therapist working in regulated organisations to make a disclosure to the police. A formal request from the police to provide information relating to the identity of a driver under the Road Traffic Act 1988 is an example. Proceeds of crime and money laundering can sometimes be another. A therapist working in private practice, on the other hand, may need to take supervisory and legal advice. Such scenarios are rare in usual practice and will likely be identified as at least *may* disclose situations in the first instance.

Circumstances in which a therapist may disclose

1. Disclosure of a 'serious crime'
2. Other public interest
3. Organisational or contractual rules, for example within your employment contract. This is the most common disclosure scenario likely to be encountered by therapists in usual practice. Here, there is a discretion conferred on the therapist, necessarily balancing competing and conflicting interests. It may not be an easy decision.

It is generally understood that private, confidential therapeutic relationships are in the public interest. The privacy of personal, sometimes intimate information goes to the heart of a trusted therapeutic relationship. The availability of therapeutic support is vital in a happy, developed environment and an important part of the well-being of society and its citizens. Arguably, never has mental health and well-being been more in the public consciousness, and the therapeutic community play a vital role.

Beyond this, a StopSO therapist may play an important, even critical role in ameliorating the risk posed by a particular person. Treatment and intervention work, with risk and harm prevention at its core, confers enormous benefits to the client, potential victims the world over and to society more generally. Although the state plays a key role in providing treatment and intervention to offenders through HM Prison and probation service, the capacity of this service has important limitations. It can only deal with persons who have been convicted of offences and where a court has passed a sentence requiring such intervention. There is often a long gap between a person who has committed offences and support from probation beginning, not infrequently a matter of years. It is a gap addressed by the private, charitable and third sector, and StopSO therapists play their part. Public resources are scarce and necessarily pointed at those where need is greatest. The intervention work of a StopSO therapist may only be part of the jigsaw, but it can be an important part.

Allied to the public interest in confidential therapeutic relationships is the private interest of the client or third parties in ensuring their privacy is maintained. Confidentiality and privacy are the starting point not least because of the high importance we attach to such confidence. Information about ourselves, especially those arising in therapeutic relationships, is likely to be intensely private and highly sensitive. Individuals who have that privacy breached might experience significant harm directly and consequently. Furthermore, they may lose faith in the therapeutic and treatment community, increasing barriers to change or driving them underground, both away from support but also from supervision and monitoring.

When considering the private rights arising in disclosure decisions it can be particularly important to bear in mind the private rights of a victim or witness. They may want their story kept private, or may prefer to tell it on their own terms at a time of their own choosing.

Disclosure of a serious crime

It is generally understood that there is a compelling public interest in detecting, preventing and prosecuting serious crime. As a society it is broadly recognised that those who do serious wrong ought to face the consequences of their actions. As citizens, therapists face the same moral dilemmas as everyone else, and no doubt experience the same range of moralised responses. Those so called 'moral' duties will vary enormously from person to person and will depend on a huge range of personal and professional experiences. Factors of community, family, faith, logic, philosophy and otherwise all feed into our system of values. Nonetheless, wherever a therapist may find themselves personally, there is no real doubt that the therapeutic community exists against a broad consensus that the public interest in detecting, preventing and prosecuting serious crime is weighty and compelling. This importance and this consensus are reflected in guidance issued by the NHS, for example, guidance echoed by many of the professional bodies regulating or supporting the therapeutic community.

Additionally, a disclosure decision may also require consideration of the private interests of an individual in the detection, prevention or prosecution of serious crime. Such crimes may have real victims. Our justice system relies on individuals doing the right thing, providing evidence to law enforcement of things they have seen or heard, often to no personal benefit and indeed often at not inconsiderable inconvenience, stress or cost. The justice system relies on this approach, but so do many victims of serious crime. They may go without justice otherwise. This may be no less true if the victim is unknown or unidentified. That is not to say that such interests are easy to know, nor that a therapist should presume or assume to know what a victim of crime would want. However, it is an important factor in the balance. Inevitably, the interests in maintaining confidentiality conflict with the interests in detecting, preventing and prosecuting serious crime. If a person tells a therapist they have committed or are contemplating committing a crime, the therapist must weigh these competing interests.

There is no clear definition of 'serious crime' but it is widely understood to potentially include sexual offences and almost inevitably includes child sexual offences. Viewing child sexual abuse material (CSAM) or communicating sexually online with or about children is likely to amount to a 'serious crime'. However, the position will not always have an easy answer. The NHS guidance says, 'serious crime will include crimes that cause serious physical harm but also include other crimes that have a high impact on the victim' (Department of Health, 2010, p. 9). This leaves many offences in an arguably uncertain category. Ultimately, the more serious the offence, the more likely it is to be necessary to disclose in the public interest, and vice versa.

Other public interest

There are various other public interests which may lead a therapist to make a disclosure. This may include disclosures about clients who may cause serious harm to others (in a way that is not a 'serious crime'). Examples include 'loophole' perpetrators (who deliberately target behaviours that are not necessarily strictly illegal, but are certainly harmful); 'gateway' perpetrators (those engaging in escalating or plainly risky, harmful behaviours, but who have not yet specifically committed an offence); those proposing to breach notification requirements; and those acting in breach of bail conditions, particularly where harm or risk is particularly elevated.

A complex and sometimes difficult topic arises when a client admits to having a sexual attraction to children (or another illegal sexual deviancy), but they claim not to have ever acted on it, nor expect to. Thoughts can never of themselves amount to a 'serious crime'. A sexual risk order requires an *act* of a sexual nature. Such a scenario would require a judgement about the necessity of disclosing to prevent a serious crime. There would be a significant element of risk assessment. There is no general public interest in knowing what a person is thinking – public interest is different from an interested public – but there does need to be a reasonable assessment of all the risk factors. Such an individual, for example, who is otherwise displaying poor coping skills, other hypersexuality and/or who has a history of working and volunteering with children might be in a very different position from a person with none of these features in their presentation. As with all of the *may* disclose scenarios, there is no general overarching duty to disclose. A therapist must weigh the competing public and private interests. Here, the public interest in preventing crime and preventing harm may be powerful, but this will only lead to disclosure if the risks are too high or unmanageable. On the other side, the interests of the client in maintaining privacy and the therapeutic relationship sit alongside the public interest in both confidential therapeutic relationships and the benefits of such a person getting potentially risk-ameliorating support.

This wider public interest may also include the topic of deliberately or recklessly spreading infectious or communicable diseases. This is a complex topic, and a therapist should seek further advice if it arises. Disclosure to the DVLA or other professional that a person is unfit to drive may also fall into this category, especially if they propose to continue driving without self-reporting. A client might be known to be using a different identity to avoid law enforcement consequences. This is distinct from where a client has changed their name lawfully for whatever reason, but might arise where a therapist learns, for example, that a client used a different persona to find work with children or vulnerable adults.

Organisational or contractual rules

A therapist may have a written contract with a client which defines additional circumstances of disclosure. A therapist might be employed in a setting, like the NHS, where the employer sets disclosure rules. Those working for the state (especially the national probation service, the local authority, police or having agreed to be a part of multi-agency public protection arrangements) will have different considerations. Additionally, the therapist may be a member of a registered body or membership organisation, where that body has rules about disclosure. Even where the therapist is not a registrant of any relevant organisation, they may feel aligned with such practice. Overall, in such cases a therapist may have to either comply with the organisational disclosure rules or leave their role or registration.

What other factors might need to be balanced in a *may* disclose scenario?

Each case will require a fact-specific balancing exercise between disclosure and confidentiality. Ultimately, it is a test of necessity and proportionality. In addition to the overarching principles discussed above, some typical factors for disclosing might be:

- Disclosure is necessary to prevent a serious crime from happening/continuing.
- Disclosure is the only way a serious crime would likely be detected.
- The crime is particularly heinous or serious.
- The harm caused by the crime is particularly serious.
- The risk to the public or specific persons if there is no disclosure is significant (for example, a known child or vulnerable adult or a person stalking a known victim).
- The risk to the public or a specific person is low, but the harm that would follow if the risk materialises is particularly significant. For example, when working with a currently low risk client who has a history of sporadic but extremely serious behaviour.
- The therapeutic work is ineffective in any event.

Some typical factors for not disclosing might be:

- Disclosure of information could not be acted upon in any event.
- The information held is too uncertain or ambiguous, like hearsay or rumor.
- The crime or harm disclosed is modest in seriousness (therapists are not obliged or expected to conduct law enforcement).
- The client interest in maintaining the therapeutic relationship is particularly strong, for example when there a client is in an action phase of intervention and disruption would be harmful.
- The public interest in maintaining privacy in therapy and treatment is particularly strong, for example, when the client is already under police investigation and they have used that as a catalyst to reach out for help.
- The police or recipient already know the information.
- Prevention, protection or risk mitigation can be achieved adequately without disclosure or with some lesser disclosure.
- The private interests of the client in maintaining confidentiality are particularly strong, for example where an individual has chosen to disclose that they were a victim of abuse and does not want to report the matter.
- The private interests of a third party are particularly strong, for example where a victim is known to have positively chosen not to report.

How does this work in practice?

Each therapist should have a privacy or data management policy and a client contract in any event. This topic falls under non-consensual disclosures of personal data or other information. A client should understand before therapy that disclosure of serious crime or serious harm may result in disclosure to the police or other authority, without their knowledge or consent if necessary. However, a therapist should always try to obtain informed consent for a disclosure, unless it is in the public interest to proceed without consent or when the therapist has already decided that they will disclose in any event. This might arise for reasons or urgency, to avoid tipping off or to protect the client or others. Generally, the client should be informed of the disclosure, unless the public interest is otherwise (for example where the client might realistically dispose of evidence). It is important for the therapist to act with honesty and candor.

It may be necessary to discuss the potential disclosure with the client to fully understand how to weigh the competing or conflicting interests. For example, a therapist might learn that the police already know of the matter through some other source. Alternatively, a client may choose to make a disclosure themselves. A common difficulty arises around the extent of knowledge or the certainty of the information. A disclosure may be partial or vague. It is not the role of the therapist to become a detective, but nor is it professional to turn a blind eye. A lack of certainty may be a factor against disclosure.

Some clients make a disclosure knowing and perhaps wanting that to lead to a law enforcement disclosure. That there are such a myriad of possible circumstances highlights the need to undertake a balancing exercise each time. There may be no clearly right answer.

Case study 1

Therapist A was supporting a client who had recently been arrested for accessing indecent images of children online. The police had seized all of his electronic devices. During police interview he had confessed to accessing illegal imagery online. He was released on bail pending the many months it would take for the police to forensically examine the content of his devices. He immediately sought support, including engaging in weekly sessions with a StopSO therapist. Progress appeared positive. He acknowledged his harmful and offending behaviours and began to show insight.

During one session, the client told the therapist that, to this great shame, he had also for some years been secretly recording his partner and another family member using a hidden camera in the bathroom. He said he had captured hours of footage of each in a state of undress, using the toilet and showering. He acknowledged that this had been for his sexual gratification. Although this offending behaviour had lasted several years he had since stopped. The last recording was more than a year prior. He had once uploaded some of the footage to an online platform on the dark web. He was still living with the partner.

The therapist had to decide whether to make a disclosure about this information to the police and/or to the partner and family member.

Although the information held by the therapist was private and confidential, the therapist had to consider the public interest in detecting, preventing and prosecuting crime, as well as the private interests of the client and victims. It appeared likely that the police were presently unaware of the offending. Whilst the police might have uncovered evidence of this voyeurism during their investigation, this was uncertain. The behaviour very likely amounted to a serious crime. The recording, retention and sharing of such images, with two victims over a sustained period indicated features of both higher harm and higher culpability. It is offending that likely had a significant impact on a victim (even if they did not yet know of it). Furthermore, the admitted diversity of offending was relevant to risk management.

On the other hand, such a disclosure to the police might significantly impact on the therapeutic relationship and the good work being undertaken. Equally, the news would no doubt be devastating for the partner and family member, and the consequences for the family unit would be enormous.

The therapist decided that it was necessary and proportionate to tell the police. The therapist decided that it would be inappropriate to tell the partner directly. The therapist concluded that the public interest in detecting and prosecuting separate offending was sufficiently high to justify breaching confidentiality, even though the offending had stopped some time ago. The potential right of the victims to know what had happened was also important. Although there was a possibility that the police would find evidence anyway, this felt too uncertain, especially relating to the time period and extent of the offending behaviour. The therapist discussed the matter with their supervisor on an anonymous basis and also with a legal helpline. They agreed that some therapists would have concluded that it was not necessary and proportionate to disclose, especially given that the offending had stopped, the intervention and therapeutic treatment appeared to be going well and that the client was already in the hands of the police. Nonetheless, for this therapist the nature and seriousness of the crime and the public interest in detecting and prosecuting such offending weighed heavily.

Case study 1 continued

The therapist decided to tell the client about the proposed disclosure. There was no imperative to withhold this from the client. The client was understanding. He said he thought this might happen but that he wanted to be frank. He asked to be given a few days so that he could find a time to tell his partner personally. He asked to continue working with the therapist, respecting their professionalism and candour.

The client told his partner the following day. She appeared to take the news well and said that she suspected him anyway. The therapist called the police officer in charge of the case the day after, and told the officer what had happened. The police were grateful for the information, but never asked for a statement. The client and therapist continued working together routinely for the following two years. He stayed with his partner, but the other family member never spoke to either of them again.

The client later pleaded guilty to various offences and received a suspended sentence order, which included requirements to attend a sex offender's programme. He was put on the sex offenders register for ten years and made subject to a sexual harm prevention order, ensuring that the police could continue to inspect his electronic devices.

A therapist should always take advice from their supervisor (see Chapter 14) or other support sources (insurance or legal helpline), albeit deploying client anonymity wherever possible. However, the decision to disclose can only ever be for the individual therapist (unless it is a *must* disclose situation). It is important to understand that reasonable, right-thinking therapists may properly come to different disclosure decisions on the same facts. A therapist should record in writing the reasons for a disclosure decision, irrespective of the outcome, including the discussion with their supervisor (and any other third party, such as insurance company or lawyer). It is best practice to record all disclosure decisions, not only those that result in a positive disclosure to a third party. Not only is the exercise itself useful, but a therapist may need to be accountable for their decision later.

The starting point is to maintain confidentiality and privacy. However, if the public and/or private interests in making a disclosure outweighs both the client interests and the public or private interest in privacy, a disclosure should be made, limited in extent to that necessary and proportionate; the disclosure would accordingly be necessary in the public and/or private interest and proportionate to the rights of the individual in privacy. Otherwise, no disclosure should be made.

Some common questions and issues

What about the public interest in a client getting help to desist from offending or harmful sexual behaviour?

Reducing the risk of offending and risk of causing harm is certainly in the public interest. If disclosing offending to the police interrupts or ruins that work or future rehabilitation work, it might be thought that greater harm flows from disclosing than not. The extent to which the therapist can reduce risk might be one of the factors in the balance. Maintaining trust with the client and in the treatment community generally will be important factors. The fact that a particular person is in the action phase of potential rehabilitation is reason to continue support. On the other hand, sexual abuse can have profound, lifelong consequences for victims and the seriousness of sexual harm cannot be overstated. How these factors weigh in an individual case will be a question for the individual therapist. Whilst it is fair and proper for a therapist to celebrate their work, it is also important not to overstate the impact with a particular client.

Case study 2

Therapist B was working with an older man. Their work had come to focus on the nature of his physical relationship with his wife during their long but recently broken marriage. He lived alone in a terraced house. His neighbours had two young female children. The client disclosed that he thought he may have recorded the children bouncing on a trampoline whilst naked. He was a keen 'twitcher' and he had been using a video camera to record an unusual bird from an upstairs window. The children were outside playing. He was unsure what he had recorded, so he deleted all of the footage without viewing it. He was troubled that he had not been more careful and that he had continued standing at the window recording even when aware he could see the children were playing naked below.

The therapist had to decide whether to make a disclosure. The client had disclosed potentially risky or troubling behaviour and was obviously concerned about the direction of his own thinking. He continued to live in close proximity to the young children.

The admitted behaviour did not appear to amount to a confession to a serious crime. It was not, on his account, a crime at all, because he did not admit that sexual gratification was a purpose of seeing or recording the children. However, there might have been a public interest in public protection policing to be aware of the issue, especially given the potential access to young children. The parents of the children might also have wanted to know about the matter, generally and to manage any risk.

On the other hand, what was known by the therapist was uncertain and vague. In reality, the police would have been unable to act on the information. The client was well engaged in therapy and this experienced therapist had a real opportunity to continue working with him, further exploring risk and undertaking any necessary intervention work. All that might well have been jeopardised by a disclosure.

Case study 2 continued

The therapist discussed the matter with their supervisor on an anonymised basis. The therapist concluded that the private interests of the client in maintaining confidentiality in the therapeutic relationship outweighed any other interests in disclosure. It was not necessary nor proportionate to make a disclosure. The therapist followed advice to make a written note of the disclosure decision, recording what was known and the different factors weighed. The therapist also told the client honestly and with candour about the issue.

What about when a client is already under police investigation or state supervision?

When the police or probation are already involved, the public interest in the detection, prevention and prosecution of crime may already be met, and so the public and private interest in maintaining a private therapeutic relationship may be pre-eminent. However, where a client discloses new offending (relapse or diversification), where they appear to present a significantly heightened risk (for example access to a child the police are not aware of) or where they disclose a serious crime which is not part of the police investigation, a fresh disclosure decision will be required. Disclosure of having perpetrated historical sexual abuse might fall into this category. Weighing the competing factors must be done afresh, remembering that although a client may confess to historical abuse, disclosure removes the right of that particular victim to choose if and when that disclosure should be made. The victim may not be ready or even wish for the offence to be disclosed. These are difficult, nuanced decisions.

How do I know if particular behaviour is a 'serious crime'?

It may not be obvious. For example, the information available to the therapist may be incomplete or uncertain. Moreover, 'serious crime' is not well defined. Firstly, consider taking legal advice based upon the best notes you have of what you have been told. Secondly, uncertainty will be an important factor when weighing the competing interests. Thirdly, you may seek further information to help inform your decision.

Would we be better off with a German style 'Dunkelfeld' support service where individuals who feel they need help can get therapeutic support without a risk of disclosure to law enforcement?

Firstly, the German Dunkelfeld system, which affects therapeutic support to individuals who express an attraction to children without breaching the person's confidentiality, is not our UK system. This chapter shows that the legal and ethical framework does allow a therapist to receive such disclosures and to keep them private, subject to a court order to the contrary, even when there is a compelling public interest in disclosure. Whether such a stance is ethical for a UK therapist will often be much more difficult: there will always be grey areas. A case by case approach is needed. Nonetheless, in reality an individual disclosing to a state-funded professional previously unknown or undetected paedophilia or admitting having accessed indecent images of children will face a significant risk of being reported to the police. No therapist, NHS, private or charitable, can promise complete privacy because they could still be ordered by a court to disclose, even if such orders are rare in practice. The same individual approaching the Dunkelfeld project would not face that disclosure risk, and the subsequent public criminalisation or associated stigma. They would get help. It seems obvious that such a person is more likely to come forward for that help, when otherwise they would remain hidden. The German-style support service might be thought to lend state support to the importance of frank disclosures in addressing unhealthy, risky or offending behaviours. The project has plainly been important in thousands of men (mainly) in Germany getting support to avoid offending or re-offending who would not have been reached otherwise. The project is unapologetic that its main aim is to protect children from being abused. Confidentiality and safe disclosures are part of that. However, even in Germany, the confidentiality is not necessarily legally absolute and it might be the broader public consensus that intervention can prevent harm to children which is central. Moreover, critics might be concerned that whilst therapeutic intervention is capable of reducing risk, in those thousands of known cases there has been a failure to allow the state to monitor and control the risks. The potential of state law enforcement agencies to join up information and to use a multi-agency approach is all lost. If the therapeutic intervention is successful then all well and good. But if it is not, the project might represent a missed opportunity for professionals to save children from serious harm.

Is there a difference between public or charitable services and private therapy?

In principle there is no difference. Those working for the NHS will be subject to NHS guidance and a charity may have its own guidance or standards. A private therapist may be subject to other memberships or accreditations, with different rules or emphasis. It is the experience of the author that those with a history of working in the public sector sometimes place greater weight on the public interest in detecting, preventing and prosecuting serious crime. They might be more likely to disclose. Those with a history in private practice might place greater weight on the importance of private therapeutic relationships. They might be less likely to disclose. This is perhaps unsurprising and merely reflects the competing nature of the different interests that arise. However, for a person seeking help the reality is uncertain and opaque, and practice may vary significantly from therapist to therapist. Even within the treatment community there is little consistency or consensus.

Conclusion

Therapists often have the privilege of hearing and receiving highly sensitive and personal information, including information that, if shared, might be used by the state to intervene necessarily and proportionately. There may be times when the therapist is obliged to share this information. However, the starting point is always that such information is private and confidential. Where a compelling public or private interest outweighs the public and private interests in confidentiality, the therapist may disclose, and may feel ethically or professionally bound so to do. There will be times when important decisions need to be made by therapists and the ethical debate with peers may not easily find consensus. Whilst the *must* disclose scenarios are non-negotiable, they are rare in practice. The *may* disclose situations create a discretion that is very personal, and it might be thought helpful to allow and respect individual therapists to follow their own ethical position, albeit within the same recognised framework. Different therapists faced with the same situation might properly come to a different conclusion.

Reference

Department of Health (2010) Confidentiality: NHS Code of Practice. Supplementary Guidance: Public Interest Disclosures. https://assets.publishing.service.gov.uk/media/5a757267ed915d6faf2b30d6/Confidentiality_-_NHS_Code_of_Practice_Supplementary_Guidance_on_Public_Interest_Disclosures.pdf.

Chapter 17

Correspondence with the criminal justice system needn't be scary

Terri Van-Leeson, Glyn Hudson-Allez (England & Wales), Sue Maxwell (Scotland) and Joan Birkmyre (Northern Ireland)

Introduction

When a person is convicted of a sexual offence, the magistrate or judge is aware of the offence *per se*, but, if a person pleads 'guilty', is not necessarily aware of the events that led up to the person committing the offence. It is for this reason that sentencing is usually adjourned for pre-sentence reports (PSRs), undertaken by the probation service. However, solicitors are becoming increasingly aware that, due to the pressure from an overburdened system, these reports may be hastily put together, or even provided orally, on the basis of a short interview with the defendant and therefore are insufficient to provide a complete evaluation of the person's case. Similarly, police forces and criminal solicitors are also becoming aware of the value of alleged offenders receiving ongoing personal therapy, not only to deal with the trauma of the arrest preventing suicidality, but to work on the issues that took them into crossing the line in the first place. As a consequence, it is becoming more common for the solicitors and/or barristers to request either a letter or a formal report for the court, for the judge to understand what led to the offence and what the individual has done to address their behaviour. This chapter provides some insight as to how to construct such a document that provides the necessary information to the court, without becoming part of the defence. We will commence with an overview for England and Wales, and then move on to specific issues for Scotland and Northern Ireland.

Letters and reports for the court may be requested by legal professionals. Whilst therapists can of course choose whether or not to respond to requests for court letters or reports, it is worth bearing in mind the positive reasons for complying with such requests. For instance, the therapist may want to be supportive of their client and the information that they can provide may prove useful in aiding the criminal justice process itself. Reasons for not complying include:

- fearfulness of damage to the therapeutic relationship,
- insufficient contact with the client in order to inform a judgement,
- fearfulness of misuse of the written material,
- the possibility of non-payment for what may be a large piece of work.

DOI: 10.4324/9781003509103-20

There is no doubt, however, that engaging in writing material such as letters and reports for legal purposes can initially feel very daunting and anxiety provoking, especially if the therapist is new to this process and has little previous experience in this particular area or doubts their competence, defined as, 'the possession of required skill, knowledge, qualification or capacity' (Webster & Springfield, 2007). This definition is a useful reminder when being asked to provide written documents for legal purposes, that qualified therapists *are* competent to give an opinion of the therapeutic work that they undertake.

Some of the anxiety that therapists feel about writing such documents is the fear of the document being made public, or that they will be called to court to give evidence. Although it is fair to say that all court documents are public documents, very few members of the public will have access to them, as mitigation documents do not tend to be made public, although a judge may read from them in court and that can be reported. However, court documents will be seen by all parties involved for both the prosecution and defence. It means that before writing anything, the therapist needs to obtain a written statement of informed consent from the client, and it is usual to send a copy of the final draft document to the client first for their consideration to check factual information, before it goes on to the court. In our experience, it is rare to be called to court, but the more clarity there is in the information you provide, the less likely you are to be called to attend, unless your information is particularly contentious.

Another consideration in making the decision whether or not to write to the criminal court, family court, parole board, or any specific regulatory body is whether or not to charge for the service, and if so, how much? Writing a letter should not take too much of the therapist's time, but a full report can be time-consuming, and it is difficult to know in advance how much reading material there will be, and how much time it will take to write. Solicitors will often ask what your fee will be before engaging you to write it, which can be tricky. It may be helpful, therefore, to offer a ballpark hourly rate, based on the hours you anticipate it will take you, highlighting it is an assessment of the hours involved rather than a specific figure that may leave you out of pocket. In our experience, reports often take longer to write than you think, but the solicitor has the choice to accept or reject your fee.

Another point to make about choosing whether to write anything for the court will depend on the quality of the notes you have kept. Some lawyers will ask for a copy of your notes, rather than a formal letter or report. Indeed, some therapists choose to write very little in their notes to prevent them from being useful to anyone else, but of course, the lawyers will not know this unless they see them. The point about this is that inaccurate, vague or illegible notes may be misinterpreted by others. An example is when a counsellor noted that his client had briefly mentioned a history of childhood abuse, but then chose to discuss a different trauma in her history in the session. The counsellor made a note of this and put a question mark beside the note as an *aide memoire* to remind him to return to this event in a future session. The prosecution council, however, challenged this and argued their interpretation was that the counsellor did not believe the client. So, the purpose of good notes is to assist in client-care: they need to be factual, consistent and accurate including the thought-processes behind the interventions used (Young & Hudson-Allez, 2005).

Where the therapist chooses to provide written material for legal purposes, it is important to be aware of the purpose in doing so and by whom this material may be read. Before providing such written material, data protection requirements mean that therapists need to carefully consider the Information Commissioner's Office (ICO) data minimisation principle. Presenting the facts is crucial throughout the written document and even though it is very difficult to avoid any unconscious bias, if the relevant facts are presented in an authentic, honest and professional non-judgemental manner, then this information can greatly assist the judicial process.

Therapeutic report vs expert witness assessment of risk

There is an important distinction to make between your input as a therapist practitioner as opposed to a risk assessor. Essentially, as a therapist practitioner you are providing the court with helpful information about what you have been doing therapeutically with the client, what areas you have explored or targeted with them in sessions, in what ways the work has addressed their sexual offending, how they have engaged, what progress you believe they have made and any recommendations to the court for either continued therapy or any other avenues of intervention you identify the client may benefit from. It is essential not to stray into areas that a court would consider not part of your jurisdiction by making comments on how risky or not you think the client is because of your work with them. There are two key reasons why you should avoid commenting at all on the level and nature of risk a client may continue to pose in terms of possible future reoffending.

The first reason is that it is considered to be wholly unacceptable for a therapist practitioner to work with a client and then *also* asses the risk of that client. It is considered that a therapist practitioner in this situation would not be able to provide an objective, unbiased opinion of the risk their client may or may not pose in the future. The argument is based on the premise that a good therapist develops a strong therapeutic working alliance with the client, becomes empathetic toward the client and validates and values the client despite some of the abusive behaviours the client may have perpetrated toward others in the past. This is essentially the role of the therapist, to value and support clients, to be non-judgemental to allow the client to explore and learn about their own difficulties that have led them to become sexually abusive toward others. So, the role of the therapist is one of support, collaborative alliance, validation and so on, and will impact on the therapist's ability to view the riskiness of the client through an unbiased lens. The approach of separating out the therapist from the risk assessor is based on the case of Anthony Rice who was a known offender, but had been released into the community partly on the recommendations of practitioners who had undertaken extensive therapeutic work with him whilst in custody. Following his release from prison, Anthony Rice went on to murder a 40-year-old woman, resulting in a serious case review (Hanson &

White, 2006). One of the many outcomes from this review included separating out the therapeutic interventionists from the risk assessors, delineating these roles to become separate and specific in order to avoid the therapeutic biases that had been evident in how practitioners had failed to objectively view Anthony Rice's continued risk toward women.

The second reason it is important to avoid commenting on how risky or otherwise a client may be is because risk assessment is a specific, specialist role that requires a variety of training. Unless you have undergone specific training in risk assessment, to include training in the use of specified structured risk assessment tools (for example the Risk of Sexual Violence Protocol-V2 (Hart & Boer, 2021)) you would be considered by a court to be operating outside of your area of expertise. Risk assessment is a specialist field. That is not to say that as a therapist you cannot enter into this area, but you would need to gain specialist supervision and undertake the relevant training. Notwithstanding the risk of recidivism assessment as a professional opinion, your discussion may include other areas of risk, such as risk of escalation, risk of diversification, risk of causing harm to oneself, risk of causing harm to others, risk of suicide and risk of deterioration of health.

Expert witness

Working in the capacity of what is referred to as an expert witness whom a court may want to hear from also carries a specific set of criteria that practitioners need to abide by. The guidelines for expert witness work set out what is required of someone who operates in this role, but also this role essentially means you need to be someone who is very significantly experienced in the area you are going to talk to the court about. It is advised that, as therapists, we steer clear of this area altogether, but it is worth knowing that some people do operate in this role on a regular basis by writing reports and being cross examined in court in regard to the specialist aspects of sexual offending behaviour, treatment and risk.

Writing the letter/report

Most commonly therapists are asked to provide written evidence of work done after a guilty plea has been entered, or the individual has been found guilty by trial. The judge will adjourn the trial for pre-sentence reports (PSRs) written by a probation officer. What is the reason for the therapist writing to the court for pre-sentencing? It could be argued that the therapist has much deeper insight into the person, as they have spent much more time with them. The judge will also be looking for mitigating issues as to whether to impose a custodial sentence onto the defendant. Sentencing council guidelines outline aggravating and mitigating factors to reduce a sentence, for example:

- no previous convictions **or** no relevant/recent convictions,
- remorse,

- previous good character and/or exemplary conduct,
- age and/or lack of maturity,
- mental disorder or learning disability, particularly where linked to the commission of the offence,
- demonstration of steps taken to address offending behaviour,
- physical disability or serious medical condition requiring urgent, intensive or long-term treatment,
- the person only played a minor role in the offence,
- ready cooperation with authorities.

Therefore, your correspondence will help the judge make a just decision. You need to be mindful, however, before writing anything, that you have seen the documentary evidence of the offence(s). This does not mean you need to see the whole court bundle, but certainly ask to view the documented charges and some of the witness statements. It is inadvisable to write information about the defendant's approach to the offence purely on the client's word.

Getting started

When writing either a letter on behalf of your client, or a full-blown report for the court, here are some practical guidelines for you to build up a template to work with, allowing you to fill out the individual details of your client each time. As a counsellor, therapist or clinical practitioner (however you label yourself) it is important to outline what your qualifications are and which governing body you are registered or aligned with (*i.e.* BACP, UKCP, COSRT or BPS). It is helpful to set out in a short summary what your experience is, and your experience of working with clients who have problems with unhealthy sexual practices and/or people who have committed sexual offences. This will be the same for all letters or reports, so can be included in your template. Letters tend to be less formal in structure, but need to clearly address the issues discussed below, and signed and dated. Matthew Graham has produced a really helpful template for a letter, which can be found in Appendix A at the end of this chapter. You may find, however, that if the therapy you have been conducting with your client has been more trauma-informed working on their historical trauma and/or abuse, that you have yet to address the offending behaviour issues that he outlines in the template. In this case, briefly outline the work that you have undertaken, but be mindful to only include detail relevant the subsequent offence.

Writing a full report

You need to consider exactly who the document is for, and why you have been asked to comment on your client. Keep this in the forefront of your mind, so that you don't start writing irrelevant information you may have ascertained through your work with your client. Reports need a formal structure, with a front page, a contents page, and an executive summary of the purpose of the report; this is a synopsis of the information you are going to provide in a short paragraph, which provides the reader with a short refresher of the whole document if they had read the whole thing through at an earlier time. It is wise to construct the provision of information clearly with paragraph headings, which are clearly numbered.

The main areas to highlight at its beginning of the report include general details of the client including name, age, gender, marital status, details of the children, living and contact arrangements with partner/spouse and children. The report provided should include details of the client's current medication, past or current addictions and any substance abuse or misuse. Other areas for consideration include details of the client's historical background where relevant, including any family history, past grief or loss, relationship history, sexual history and especially any disclosure of past abuse /sexual abuse, although you need to be mindful of the confidentiality aspect of this and only include it if it is relevant.

Then it is helpful to the court if you set out what your involvement with the client has been, from the point of referral, assessment, duration of therapy and the progress made to date if you are still working with them. It is also important to provide information regarding attendance/non-attendance dates for therapy together with an overall therapeutic/psychological assessment which gives details of any neurodivergence, the client's health and especially their mental health, as very often these clients can be at risk of potential for suicide. Providing brief details of the work done in therapy, for example, work on relapse prevention, victim empathy work and remorse noted is also very relevant, demonstrating they have taken steps to address offending behaviour and have a treatment pathway. Rehabilitation needs to be deemed as a realistic prospect, or may have already been conducted in the long wait before sentencing.

The report should include the specific questions that you have been asked to address from the client's solicitor, copied into the report, with clear answers that stay with the point of the question. You will need to provide references for any expressions of opinion that you have gleaned from the literature, or if it is your personal opinion, you need to say so and how you evidence your inference. It is also important to be shown to be unbiased by including any literature that does not support your opinion.

In concluding the written document, a paragraph outlining the therapist's future recommendations can provide details of benefit from any further work, therapy or referral to any other appropriate agencies. However, whatever information you provide, be objective, unbiased and dispassionate using a measured independent tone, providing reasons for the opinion that you have reached. You are allowed to change your opinion if evidence subsequently materialises that you were not aware of, but it must be done promptly. Do not lose sight of the fact that this report is written for the benefit and understanding of the court, not to provide your client with a defence. Formal reports usually end with a statement to this effect and that you have not been asked to amend your report in any way. Some solicitors may ask you to do this, but it essential that you stay with your own opinion of the client, and not be persuaded to change that opinion by anyone else. Your final sentence should be an assurance that you have told the truth as you understand it.

Sometimes it is helpful to include appendices in a formal report, which may include your CV, references, a glossary of therapeutic/psychological terms and a list of the papers read from the court bundle. In writing such reports, it is always useful to remember that less is more; the more you write, the less the reader will take in. Also remember the primacy and recency effect: people remember more about the beginning and end of your document than they will the middle, which is why your initial summary at the beginning and your overview in the conclusion are so important.

The above guidance is based on the requirements of England and Wales. Being mindful that other areas of the United Kingdom have different legislative requirements, there follows sections referring specifically to Scotland and Northern Ireland.

Scotland

England and Wales employ a binary verdict system of guilty or not guilty. Scotland, however, retains a three-verdict system comprising guilty, not guilty and not proven. The not proven verdict is unique to Scottish law and means that the evidence presented did not establish guilt beyond reasonable doubt. It is not a pronouncement of innocence. However, similarly, the not guilty verdict in England Wales is not a finding of fact that the defendant did not do it, it is merely a finding that the jury could not be sure that the defendant did what was alleged. In Scotland, jury-less trials and/or single judge trials to speed up processing rape and sexual assault cases was mooted in April 2024. By October 2024, the idea had been abandoned by the government following discussion with victim groups, legal colleagues and human rights groups etc.

In Scotland, internet sexual offence cases are dealt in the Sheriff Court. The Procurator Fiscal presents the case for the prosecution to the Sheriff and the defence solicitor for the person accused. The accused may have been directed via a flyer given out at point of arrest to the Lucy Faithfull Foundation (previously Stop it Now Scotland) and/or to have looked for a therapist via StopSO or other organisations. They may also have been signposted to see their GP because of the distress they feel. During the ensuing 18 months to two years, it is best if the accused, who becomes a client, embarks on understanding their actions that led to the alleged offence and makes appropriate behaviour changes.

Once the forensic evidence of the person is seen by prosecutor, defence solicitor and Sheriff, he is formally charged and may plead guilty at this time. The Sheriff asks for reports from the criminal justice social (CJS) work department and gives a date for sentencing in five to eight weeks. These reports usually take between one and one and a half hours to conduct, and assess the level of risk the accused presents, referring to sentencing guidelines of the Sexual Offences Act 2003. That report is sent to the Sheriff and usually the prosecutor and the defence solicitor. The client may not know until the day of sentencing what the report says.

As a therapist I may have met the client for ten to 20 sessions, so I will write a report for the defence team with the client's consent. The client will have seen the therapist's report in advance of the sentencing date. Stop it Now will also present a report about the Group Work the client has participated in. The Sheriff, prosecutor and defence council share all reports, while the Sheriff sentences.

A contact offence, rape and sexual assault and more extreme sexual crimes go to the High Court and are heard by a judge. The defence in these cases usually engage a barrister to present the case in court. There is a possibility that in the future in Scotland, rape cases may be handled differently, but there is much debate at present (2024) amongst affected survivors, lawyers and policy makers about this.

Northern Ireland

In Northern Ireland, sex offenders are managed according to the Sexual Offences (Northern Ireland) Order 2008.These laws outline similar procedures and regulations to those in Scotland and England but there may be differences in specific details and implementation due to variations in the legal systems and policies between the regions. Once someone is convicted of a sexual offence in Northern Ireland, they will be risk assessed by psychologists and then according to the judge's verdict, they are usually recommended towards an appropriate treatment programme managed by the Probation Board N.I. These programmes have been designed according to the risk level of the offender, *i.e.* low, medium or high, and are delivered in small groups usually of around eight to ten people, but sometimes work of a one-to-one nature may also be offered.

In comparison to procedures elsewhere in the United Kingdom, the police service of Northern Ireland are unlikely to refer individuals for therapy prior to their sentencing, which may be a missed opportunity for alleged sexual offenders to have in-depth individual therapy to establish the root causes of their behaviour and to look at the possibility of rehabilitation and reducing the risk of reoffending. To date there are six therapists, including myself, working on behalf of StopSO in Northern Ireland. Clients are generally referred directly to us and the majority of them are usually in the early investigative stages of their offences. Some clients may also self-refer or solicitors may recommend individual therapy to them. Not all professionals/organisations who work with sexual offenders or their partners are aware of this as a possible worthwhile course of action, or are even knowledgeable about StopSO-trained Therapists in Northern Ireland.

Solicitors in Northern Ireland tend to ask for evidence of attendance at therapy, with the individual's consent. Court reports written by the therapist can provide more helpful detail and evidence on behalf of the client and thus contribute to more informed court decisions. Therapists undertaking this work need to have access to good supervisors who are trained in this field of work. Supervision, whilst being essential, is also helpful in preventing vicarious trauma, which can sometimes occur given its difficult nature (see Chapter 14). The supervision can also be beneficial in assisting the therapist towards being competent in providing such written material for legal purposes. It is also worth bearing in mind, that from a legal perspective, sentencing guidelines take into consideration the realistic prospect that people may take demonstrable steps to address their offending behaviour and where this is the case, then mitigating factors can apply. In my work as a StopSO therapist, this fact has influenced my past decisions in whether to provide the relevant information to legal bodies for some past clients who have committed sexual offences. Also, the feedback given to me from previous clients suggests that the therapy has proved beneficial as it has helped them to understand the root causes of their harmful behaviour and work towards changing this, especially with a view to establishing more healthy relationships including healthy sexual behaviour. This, of itself, is rehabilitation and hopefully leads to the reduction in the risk of reoffending.

References

Graham, M. (2024) StopSO Writing letters for Court. Law and Practical Guidance for StopSO Therapists. Webinar, 4 June 2024.

Hanson, D. & White, E. (2006) An Independent Review of a Serious Further Offences case. HM Inspectorate of Probation. https://www.justiceinspectorates.gov.uk/probation/wp-content/uploads/sites/5/2014/03/hansonandwhitereview-rps.pdf.

Hart, S. D.& Boer, D. P. (2021) Structured professional judgment guidelines for sexual violence risk assessment the sexual violence risk-20 (svr-20) versions 1 and 2 and Risk for Sexual Violence Protocol (RSVP). In K. S. Douglas & R. K. Otto (eds) *Handbook of Violence Risk Assessment*. 2nd ed. Routledge. doi:10.4324/9781315518374.

Information Commissioner's Office (n.d.) Principle C: Data minimisation. https://ico.org.uk/for-organisations/uk-gdpr-guidance-and-resources/data-protection-principles/a-guide-to-the-data-protection-principles/the-principles/data-minimisation/.

Sentencing Council Guidelines (n.d.) Aggravating and mitigating factors. https://www.sentencingcouncil.org.uk/explanatory-material/magistrates-court/item/aggravating-and-mitigating-factors/.

Webster, M. & Springfield, M. A. (2007). Merriam-Webster's Dictionary and Thesaurus. Google Scholar. https://scholar.google.com/scholar?q=Webster+M+Merriam-Webster%27s+Dictionary+and+Thesaurus+Springfield,+MA+Merriam-Webster,+Inc.+2007+.

Young, T. & Hudson-Allez, G. (2005) *Writing reports and giving evidence in court. A guide for psychological therapists.* Counsellors and Psychotherapists in Primary Care Monograph 6: Court.

Appendix A

Example StopSO Reference for a Criminal Court (Graham, 2024)

HEADED PAPER

[full title, full name]
[professional organisation if applicable]
[correspondence address]
[email]
[contact number
[date]

Dear Judge,

I am a professional [therapist/counsellor] and have been working with [the defendant]. I am providing this document in respect of his forthcoming sentencing hearing.

Introduction

I have been in professional practice for [..] years. As part of my regular professional practice I work with individuals who have sought help in respect of harmful sexual behaviours, including those who are accused or who have committed sexual offences, whether online, in person or otherwise. Over the course of my professional practice I have worked with [dozens/hundreds/numerous/various] such cases and my current caseload includes [many/a number] of such cases. I also work with victims and survivors of sexual abuse, as well as family members and non-offending partners involved in these cases.

I am a member of StopSO UK, a specialist treatment organisation for perpetrators and survivors of sexual offending. I am also a member of [ATSAC/UKCP/ BPS/BACP] and further details of my professional qualifications and experience can be found at Appendix One and further details of these organisations and affiliations at Appendix Two.

Work with [defendant name]

I began work with [defendant name] in [month and year]. We had our first session on [date] and have been meeting [weekly/fortnightly/monthly] since. In total we have had [number of sessions] each of [duration of session]. The work is [ongoing/

currently paused/completed]. Our work has been conducted [in person/by video call/combination]. In total [defendant's name] has spent over [total hours] in personal one-to-one treatment.

Overall assessment
[Defendant's name] has engaged [conscientiously and consistently] throughout our time together. He has [never missed an appointment]. Although he [was obviously in crises/highly anxious] in the early phase of our work, he presents as having committed himself to a change process. [I have been impressed with his willingness to confront his unhealthy and offending habits with a commitment to sustainable desistence/He has found it hard to confront his demons, but has persisted and shown a willingness to be challenged]. He has [worked hard/done his best/kept going], completed various additional tasks outside of our therapy sessions and in my observation [has confronted many of the underlying factors his formerly harmful behaviours/has the potential to get benefit from further work / would benefit from continuing support].

[Other agencies/Other work]
[defendant's name] work with me has not been in isolation. I understand that he has also completed the [Lucy Faithful Inform Plus Course/Safer Lives Programme/Circles/Other therapy/Relate] and this has been [complimentary/additional] to our work together. Before starting with me he had completed the Stop it Now online modules and had begun reading several course texts, including [My Brain on Porn]. This wider engagement in risk reduction work, both professionally and on a self-help basis, is encouraging and commendable, giving a [defendant's name] a wider perspective and allowing a greater depth of intervention.

[Psychological Assessment of Treatment Need/Risk Assessment/Psychiatric Assessment]
I am aware that [defendant's name] was assessed by [Dr] in [month and year] and I have seen a copy of their [assessment/risk assessment/report]. This has been a useful additional tool in informing our work. The topics of [ACE/Abuse/PTSD/Addiction/Mental Health/Neurodivergence] were particularly important features. I have seen the recommended [treatment plan/treatment factors/work required] and I can confirm that [all/some/none] of these issues [have been addressed during therapy/are ongoing/remain outstanding]. I have personally spoken to [Dr] on various occasions regarding [defendant's name] to ensure that my work with him has covered the most important areas.

[Risk Focussed Work]
When [defendant's name] first began work he was in crises, expressing suicidal ideation and understandably at a very low ebb. Medication he was prescribed by his GP appeared to be of limited effect, but over time he was able to stabilise, and being able to continue to support his family appeared a major driver. From that

base we have been able to focus more on the drivers of his harmful and ultimately offending behaviours. The detail of that work is beyond this reference, but important topics have included his very low self-esteem, developed in particular during adolescence when he was bullied by his peers and his parents split, leaving him isolated and resentful. He was unsuccessful socially and confused in his sexual identify, increasingly turning to the internet. What appears to have become an addiction to pornography developed, something that he had been exposed to in the home environment before secondary school. He has described to me a growing desensitisation to mainstream pornography. This, coupled with his social isolation meant he found comfort in online group chats where increasingly extreme and illegal material was shared. [defendant's name] has not sought with me to deny or minimise his offending and this acceptance has allowed me to bring appropriate challenge to our work. I am satisfied that our work has and continues to be appropriately risk-focussed.

[Victim of Sexual Abuse – NB be careful regarding confidentiality]
[defendant's name] has disclosed to me that he has been the victim of sexual abuse. He has told me this happened during his childhood and early teens at the hands of a close family member. It has become evident to me that these experiences have had and continue to have a profound impact on [defendant's name]. Every experience is different, but those who are abused may develop a distorted view of sexual experience, with strong feelings of guilt, shame and hurt. We have begun to explore these themes in therapy and the work is ongoing.

[Remorse]
[defendant's name] has presented as remorseful for his behaviour repeatedly during our sessions together. He has been frequently tearful, expressing at times an overwhelming sense of shame and guilt. [I assess this remorse as genuine]. Having worked with many men in a similar situation over the years I am conscious that remorse for offending may be distinguished from self-pity and the burden of the consequences of having been detected and criminalised. These consequences are heavy for [defendant's name]. [However, [defendant's name] goes further, and has described waves of remorse for the victims portrayed in the images he sought, demonstrating an understanding of the harm he has caused by being a part of this recording of abuse.] [I assess this remorse as both genuine and protective for the future.]

[Homework]
[Defendant's name] has consistently engaged in a variety of home learning I have recommended, in addition to our sessions together. This has included, as examples, working through the Internet Watch Foundation's 'Pixels from a Crime Scene' podcast, which he described as, 'incredibly powerful, really bringing home the awful impact on the children', personal diary keeping, writing an imagined letter to his future self, producing a weekly internet use chart. This additional work is valuable of itself, but also in my judgement demonstrates a commitment to change.

[Relapse prevention]
We have reached a point in our work where [defendant's name] has been able to develop a carefully considered relapse prevention plan. This includes careful consideration of [his circle of safety, key red flags with association actions and some quite detailed scenario planning]. I am aware that he has shared this plan with his [partner/social services/brother]. [This work has included a detailed review of his offence formulation, including the key precipitating, perpetuating and protective factors in his case.]

Mental health / Neurodivergence
[defendant's name] has been diagnosed with [PTSD/autism/ADHD/depression]. I am aware that he receives prescribed medication from his GP. [defendant's name] presents as withdrawn. He often avoids eye contact. I have found it important not to overwhelm him with information, but keep sessions structured and topic focussed. I observe that have 40 mins or so of a session his concentration will wane. He is prone to catastrophising, but we have made progress in this regard. I am mindful that he was assessed by [Dr]. His ability to engage with people he has never met before is very hard for him. If I compare his engagement with me now compared to our early sessions there is a marked difference. This may be relevant to professionals engaging with [defendant's name] now. He is capable of considerable insight and introspection, but I have observed that this can sometimes be masked by a dismissive or arrogant presentation. This characteristic may be connected to his learnt behaviours from his upbringing, of not talking about emotions, of achievement being dominant.

[Future work]
My work with [defendant's name] is, subject to his liberty, expected to continue. There remain topics relating to [self-esteem/pre-occupation/managing conflict/shame and guilt/grief] which would, in my professional assessment, benefit from further work, as well as ensuring that his exit from regular therapy is effectively and properly managed when the times comes. Subject to any order of the court, how this is undertaken may well involve liaison with a probation officer.
 I trust that this is of assistance.

Yours sincerely
[signature]

[therapist name]
[date]

Chapter 18

The last word

A client's voice

'Matt'

'Matt' came to a StopSO therapist after his release from prison after serving six years. He had previously been married with three children. He now lives alone. His story is told in his own words.

History

A biography of a traumatic life.

Traumatised children grow into traumatised adults.

Trauma. A blow that damages. An experience that is emotionally and psychologically damaging. Scar tissue is sometimes left behind as a visible sign of past trauma or damage.

Invisible trauma is not as apparent. Often the only symptoms are emotional and psychological, which can be temporarily hidden, suppressed or transformed into something else, *i.e.* acting out. For me, it would be easier to be a mass of scar tissue. At least then it would be fairly obvious how much damage had been done. The world truly has no idea of what it was like for me.

For me, it emerged as cruelty, a sadistic streak. Even at a very young age. It happened to me. I suppose if what you see is adults being cruel to you, a powerless child, vulnerable, weak . . . Well then that is what I learned to do. That it was natural. Somehow, kindness and compassion, real value for others, became a weakness to be either exploited, abused or humiliated. It happened to me. Groomed to say 'fine' when asked how things are/were. Boys don't cry.

Mum was weak. Mental and emotional ill-health. An embarrassment. A drug addict, prone to alcoholic binges, massive mood swings, intense emotional and physically violent outbursts. Not a bad person, not evil, just extremely traumatised herself. I think it's termed 'generational trauma': damage and hurt that is transmitted from one generation to the next. My grandfather sexually abused my mother and my aunt. Mum's nickname amongst her acquaintances was 'Madmags'. It was just her and me growing up. Dad was never at home. Always working away in different parts of the country. So mum was left alone with me. I didn't know anything else, so to me it was my 'normal'.

DOI: 10.4324/9781003509103-21

I was, by all accounts, what was called a 'colicky baby'. I guess I was (still am) gastro-sensitive. Generally sensitive. Light, noise, food, texture everything is very overwhelming for me (autistic sensory sensitivity?). As a baby I did what uncomfortable babies do – I cried! My mum couldn't manage. The responsibility, the noise, all of it. Still a child herself at 22 years old and full of generational trauma. The bottom fell out of my mum's world when the reality of motherhood and life became apparent. Managing money, a flat, a baby, all of it, drove my mum into a depression. Absent Dad. Unsupportive grandparents, who were delighted in saying, 'I told you so' – increased the pressure on my mother. Unsurprisingly, she turned to medication to help her cope. This quickly escalated to a full-on habit.

Mum would throw parties with lots of adults. I remember being passed around. I didn't understand what was going on, but I felt very scared and wanted my mum. Mum would ignore me and other people would hold me. I didn't want them, I wanted mum. I would pay for it later. When everyone was gone, mum would beat me, or lock me away or shout and scream and call me horrible things until I went quiet. I wasn't allowed to make a single noise. Then I would be alone. I would be crying and saying sorry. I didn't understand why I acted out, or even that I *was* acting out. I couldn't communicate how I felt. I would be in bed. Couldn't sleep. Nowhere to go or comfort me. Nothing. Then the next day, mum would make a fuss of me, everything would be wonderful, and the sun came out and it was perfect for a little while. She was my beautiful mum and I was her special little boy. We would dance and sing and play, but it never lasted.

As time passed, I remember becoming aware of a heavy feeling in my stomach and heart, it never went away, always there. No one will ever know what it was like. I lived in a permanent state of fear, then happiness, then fear, then guilt, then confusion. And always the anxiety, the sadness.

It was only as I started to see other people's lives that I began to feel shame and anger, loss and bitterness for what others appeared to have; and for what I did not. I couldn't fit into other people's lives as myself. My feral/challenging coping strategies/behaviour made me difficult and precocious. I was dramatic, wild, unpredictable, bright, energetic and creative. Gifted in many ways, but not in the ways my family supported.

School was a nightmare for me. Not understanding the school system, the other kids, not fitting in, being laughed at and ridiculed, bullied, punished for my energy, punished for not being interested. I lived in a fantasy world most of the time, my ethics and honour system and communication version of the world was very far removed from the normal school day. I would just go to school, do my best to survive the day. Other kids seemed to make friends, be in groups, understand each other and what was going on. Me, not a clue. Never got it right. Wrong clothes, wrong shoes, wrong words, wrong everything. I couldn't get on at school. The other kids confused me, I couldn't cope with the institution, the rules. I was unpredictable, angry one day, passive the next, well behaved another. Every report . . . 'good potential . . . must try harder'. So, the things I did well in, well, it felt like they were never recognised or encouraged.

I was nearly always bruised for one reason or another. At school, we would get changed for PE. The teachers noticed the bruises around my arms, body and legs. They were partly from mum (and dad when he was around) and from vigorous play. The school asked me where the bruises came from. I didn't answer, but went home and told mum. She asked me if I was being bullied at school. Was that where the bruises were coming from? This was confusing, because actually they were coming from her when she hit me, daily. But she told me I was getting bullied by nasty children at school, and so I must stand up to the bullies and tell the teacher. So I did. But I couldn't provide names, because the bullying didn't exist. So the school decided to take me from class to class, and show my bruises to the other children as an example of what happens when we are bullied. That was strange. I don't know how I felt, but I'm pretty sure I wasn't happy. Somehow, I internalised the idea of keeping my mum protected.

My life continued, mum getting worse, more abusive. Dad would turn up every now and again and pretty much ignore me. He would either be asleep in a chair, or just a pair of legs poking out from underneath his car on the front forecourt. I would collect things that belonged to him. A scarf, a glove, a shoe. I would smell them and they smelt like him. I had a little pile at the bottom of my wardrobe. He would get angry sometimes when he couldn't find something, come storming into where I slept and shout and then kick me.

Mum and Dad had always had big arguments, but they were getting worse. They had started hitting each other, things getting thrown about and smashing. Night after night. Often, I would hear them in the distance, shouting. They would get closer and closer, until they were outside my bedroom door. I could hear them hitting each other. Shouting. Then my door would burst open. Mum would come flying in her face bloody, or naked, shouting and screaming at me to please help her. Dad would follow her in, grab her, drag her out, screaming. I felt like I should have helped mum, but dad was so scary I was terrified to do anything. I just lay there, crying, waiting for them to go away. I was in such fear. I would go to bed in fear of what would happen that night. I did not sleep much. I was so scared to leave the room, When I wanted to go to the toilet, I took to weeing in the corner.

My family just thought I was a problem child, precocious, a daydreamer. No real interest in the things they wanted for me. I was an embarrassment and a disappointment. Flaky. Second rate. My Nan would even tell me how disappointed in me she was. Why couldn't I be the way she wanted? She could support me then, but not the silly dreams and worthless things I was good at, like music and art.

Over the course of my childhood, I unfortunately developed into an individual without any real sense of self-worth or self-esteem. In fact, I grew to despise myself for what I had been taught, which was that my nature and way of being was wrong. Self-destructive and mentally ill, but with some intelligence, I soon learnt to hide my feelings away. To pretend to such a degree that others did not or could not suspect how different I felt my mind and behaviour was. I hid away from the entire world, Those I loved, my wife, friends . . . everyone. I absolutely believed without a shadow of a doubt that I would be abandoned, humiliated, punished etc. if the world realised what I was really like.

I struggled to work or commit. Eventually, after many traumatic experiences, I mustered the strength to go through college. Masking the whole way. My whole life was a mask, a pretence. I did well, and eventually get a very good job. I met my ex-partner, got married. Got a mortgage. Had kids. My job involved a lot of time alone, and was a role that allowed me to hide behind a veneer of professionalism.

Self-reflection

I feel like the monster created by Doctor Frankenstein. I often feel like I've never really had a chance to flourish. Not through anyone's fault, but simply through misunderstanding and fear. Not regarded as being worthwhile for myself, only ever a blank screen for others to project onto. Do humans even see each other at all? I wonder, are we all just trying to communicate and relate to what we see as versions of ourselves? An endless mirror image?

I am not you. My experience of this world is very different from yours. I have my own perceptions, experiences, hopes. But I have been taught that they aren't worthy of love, of your attention. Not unless I accept your views of me, do nothing to threaten those views of the world as other, as yourself. I suffer all the time; I express it in various ways. Talking, music. I have learnt that things can be both light and heavy, easy and hard. That I suffer all the time, yet also at the same moment experience joy too. That is my experience.

I stopped sharing my experiences and thoughts a long time ago, when I was met either with silence, hostility or ridicule. Very, very, few people, I feel, have accepted me as I am. And I have felt a measure of safety and belonging with these people. And so I opened up. But then the fear of rejection, being ridiculed, paranoia, hurt, has kicked in and I have acted to push them away. Easier for me that way. Lonely though. Feeling constantly belittled, or dismissed, or hurt, or let down. Or judged. Or in need of fixing, improving, repairing, a charity case. Messed up, flaky. A wrong un, a monster. Evil. No good. All internalised, I feel.

Bad, wrong, warped, unlovable. Rotten at the core. After all, that is what I must be, to feel the things I do, the encompassing anger and rage at everyone and everything, and most of all, at myself for being this weak, useless, wrong, unwanted creature. Utter self-loathing. What do I do about it? Where should I have begun? I couldn't even express what I was experiencing. Such a confusing, jumbled up tumbling internal landscape, mentally and emotionally constantly living in fear, hypervigilant. And scared to talk about it for fear of repetition of the past experiences.

I literally *am* Frankenstein's Monster. . . . You see, the other side of the monster, the love, the kindness, the loyalty, the need to give and receive love feels like it was never valued, overshadowed in my mind by the monster that lived inside and would emerge, to act out, lash out, hurt those I loved and ultimately, myself.

Eventually I broke and completely stopped functioning in a reasonable way. Symptoms of depression and anxiety. Medication. We had moved to a new part of the country and I was isolated. My partner was out of her depth. I now realise that I also had complex PTSD from all the traumatic experiences I experienced. Night terrors, anger issues, risk-taking, depression, crippling anxiety, self-doubt and confusion. Constant emotional triggers would shut me down multiple times daily.

And the guilt! Terrible father, terrible husband, useless, worthless, can't work, selfish etc. etc. I couldn't describe what I was experiencing: isolation, frustration. I got worse. I just wanted my life to end. I couldn't live any sort of life; too scared to die, I existed in a foggy haze, prescription and over the counter medication to numb me enough so I could do the bare minimum . . . Which became less and less.

Offending

I found myself hating and resenting the world, people, society. I blamed them all. All the happy, normal people. Despised them. Was jealous. I desperately wanted to fit in, to be normal, to be accepted, loved, approved of. To escape and distract from these unbearable emotions was the only way I felt I could cope; addictions followed, several spiralling into each other. Eventually, lost, angry, confused, broken, alone, isolated . . . unable to express myself or even explain what was going on, I found myself compulsively watching adult porn. For hours on end, at night, when my partner and kids had gone to bed.

I slept on the couch. My night terrors meant I could be violent while asleep. I had punched and kicked my partner while experiencing these nightmares, so took to sleeping alone where I couldn't hurt anyone. Standard porn stopped being effective, and I sought out darker niches involving various types of emotional and physical abuse, eventually finding myself looking at CSAM. Even this CSAM eventually stopped being effective. I needed more risk. More power, more thrill. I graduated to a contact offence.

I had pressed the self-destruct button without thought, care or consequence. It was madness at that moment. I simply did not care, did not feel anything other than the need to escape, to feel the thrill, via the compulsion to feel powerful at that moment via the thrill of abuse. It felt like a secret power that the world knew nothing about. A sticking two fingers up to the world that I hated. Psychologically and emotionally I was a complete mess. No balanced individual abuses another. It was a sign of a deep self-hatred, in my case. I believe my desensitisation to the act through repeated viewing of CSAM also played a big part in the offence.

The knock

Arrested. They had been waiting for me. The child abuse unit officers. My wife had called me and told me the police were waiting for me and wouldn't leave. They had a warrant for my arrest. They hadn't told her why. I said I'd be home asap. I knew my life was over. I hadn't truly considered how it would affect my family. As I pulled up to the parking area at home, a silver car blocked me in. Four men got out of the car and approached me. They identified themselves as plain-clothed police officers from the Police Child Abuse Unit. They confirmed my identity and then arrested me on suspicion of rape of a child under the age of 13. They seized my phone immediately. I asked if I could enter the house and see my wife, they said I could, but not the children as they were under 18.

As I entered, my wife was standing in the front room, crying. The police asked for all the internet-enabled devices in the house to be handed over. Not just mine, but my wife's, the kids, the business PC. Everything. Phones, tablets, iPads, the lot. It was all potential evidence. I wasn't allowed to change my clothes, again, potential evidence. I was allowed to give my wife a hug. I whispered 'I'm sorry' in her ear. And said goodbye.

I wasn't allowed to see the kids. Two were upstairs in their bedroom. I didn't see them. My son was standing at the top of the stairs, crying. I couldn't approach or speak with him. That was the last time I saw my son. He was 11 years old. The police led me from the house and into the silver car. As we drove away, I looked back at the house. There at the window were the three children, all crying. That was the last I ever saw of my three children. That is the memory, the image that haunts me. I have nightmares about it, reliving it again. I wake up crying and in a state. It is so painful to write about now, even after several years. Knowing how much suffering and anguish I caused for them all. Truly, truly horrendous.

Following my appearance in the national media, my family was subject to threats and abuse. They had to be escorted by the police from home at one point as it was deemed unsafe for them to remain there. The kids were police escorted into school in the mornings, and home afterwards. My wife was left without friends. The kids were left without friends and were subject to bullying and harassment online, out in public and at school. Their lives as they knew them were utterly devastated.

The business collapsed. Government benefits were barely enough to live on. The kids and my wife needed trauma therapy. Social services became involved with the kids. There was the suggestion of my wife losing the children, as at first she tried to support me. Unless she cut me off from herself and the children, social services would consider her an unfit parent and put the children into care. My wife became a pariah. Subject to abuse, harassment, threats. Their lives were threatened. They lived in utter terror and were scared to leave the house. People that we had considered as good friends cut her off and even joined in with the abuse. Graffiti was sprayed on the house, paint thrown on the car. Stones at the windows, shit through the letterbox. I struggle to live with the thoughts of it even now, seven years later, especially as I know how deeply this has scarred them all, how much it has affected their childhood, their development. I stole their childhood from them by committing my offences. How do I live with it? Painfully. Regretfully. Guiltily. Ashamed.

Prison: self-loathing

It is like a knife twisting in my heart every time I think of it. It doesn't get easier. Because my family still suffer even after all this time. They carry the stigma of my crimes. Always will. I know they are angry and hate me for what I did. There is a very high chance I will never, ever have any sort of reconciliation with them.

My wife divorced me. Changed her and the kids' names. The children are all strangers to me now. I wouldn't recognise them if I saw them. At my arrest, they were between the ages 11 and four. They not only lost their father, but my actions caused them direct harm. They were also my victims as they suffered and continue to suffer as a consequence. Hard to live with does not do it justice.

I wish I had asked for help. Reached out and faced my demons. Nothing could be worse than the result of what happened to my family (and my victim). Most of my extended family, aunts, uncles, cousins, nieces and nephews, turned on me. My only brother turned his back on me and we have not spoken in seven years. Devastation, isolation. Self-destruction in extremis. I should have got help. The price was too high for not reaching out.

In prison, I underwent one-to-one work with a psychiatric practitioner. She was experienced working with neurodivergent individuals, and by this time I had realised that I needed to really open up and share the deepest of my fears and secrets in order to move away from the self-hatred and self-destruction. I had to admit how bad things were in order to address them. I had to face the pain of the loss of my wife and children, my extended family, friends, life, everything. It was on my knees that I realised I couldn't continue running away from myself, my trauma, my pain, shame, feelings so painful I had buried them deeply away. But they have a habit of coming back out when something triggers me. Then I would relive those moments, those experiences, those traumas I had so desperately denied and hidden away.

Neurodivergence

The psychiatrist stated that in her opinion there was a high likelihood I was on the autistic spectrum, but very high masking. This was news to me. We began working on the issues from a different perspective, one of that of a neurodivergent individual. My needs were different, my reactions and perspective on the world were very different from neurotypical individuals. The repetitive behaviours (known as Stimming) that I had suppressed now were seen as part of my autism, not just me being 'wrong'. I began to understand and accept myself . . . A tiny bit.

I have spent almost 51 of my 52 years on this planet as an *un-diagnosed* neurodivergent person. I have AuDhd. Autism and ADHD in combination.

What does that statement mean? Well, most of the difficulties I experience (sensory, social, communication, self-esteem, behavioural, mental health, C-PTSD etc.) can be attributed to being neurodivergent in a world that is *not* suited to me. Expectations put on me by my family and society were not helpful to my development. Back in the 1970s (I was born in 1972) autism/ADHD was pretty much unheard of. And mental illness and neurodivergent conditions were heaped together and treated as an affliction visited upon the weak, broken and useless. So people just got on with their lives. Bent themselves into positions where they could function. Now called masking.

Those that couldn't mask well, or just couldn't function appropriately, were left without meaningful support or understanding. The mental health hospitals were filled with the unwanted, the autistic, the mad and the bad. Drug and alcohol abuse were (and still are) common as a way to cope for those who couldn't function or understand why and how they were different. The shame and stigma associated with poor mental health and behavioural differences that went against the normal expectations was borne by the nearest and dearest to the individual, if they had any family left speaking to them by that point. So many neurodivergent individuals grew up being shamed, punished and humiliated for their differences. Not necessarily from a desire to cause harm, but to try to fix or mend, to somehow excise the neurodivergent and make us palatable to others. To fit in, and therefore to avoid the pain and humiliation we would inevitably face in the world.

My experience was exactly like this.

Being high-functioning neurodivergent did have some benefits: I am by nature honest, focussed and committed. I pushed myself to excel in everything I did, mostly to compensate for my feelings of worthlessness. I kept myself to myself, and was considered aloof, shy, weird. But my work performance and in other aspects of my life was high enough for people to overlook my oddness. Not sustainable though! Masking is exhausting and regularly leads to burnout and meltdowns. All this masking required a lot of down time to recover from. Sadly, my family paid the price, as I was not capable of being a consistent parent, husband, friend. More feelings of guilt and worthlessness feeding the spiralling self-destructive self-hatred. A lifetime in fact.

Late diagnosis

Now I know, I am on the autistic spectrum with processing, social and communication delays and issues. I have ADHD with its concomitant issues. I experience complex PTSD from all the bad experiences, heightened by my AuDhd, a kind of a triple whammy of sensory and emotional overwhelm. Acting out, not understanding neuroliteral cues, communication, norms and expectations. Punished for it my whole life. Not even knowing *what* I felt or why, or how to express it. Now known as alexithymia. All of it was missed. I received zero support or help. In fact, I was blamed, disliked and punished for the way I was. I didn't know any other way to be; I was a child on the autistic spectrum, with a highly dysfunctional family life in the 1970s. Autism? What the hell is that? Emotionally challenged, naughty, precocious, spoiled were the terms used then.

But, for the first time ever, I felt some hope of achieving a measure of self-acceptance for the real me, not the pretend me I had worked so hard to create and maintain, while the real me slowly despaired of ever seeing the light or love of being accepted. Following my prison sentence, I knew I needed to continue the work that had started. I needed to develop, to heal, to understand, to learn self-acceptance and to get to know who I really was, having shied away from my neurodivergency for my entire life.

On my release, I contacted the NHS wellbeing service and explained my situation. Sadly, they could not help me. They did not have the resources nor the experience to do so. But they did signpost me to some charities that work in the field of survivors of sexual abuse (because I was abused as a child), but unfortunately, as I am also a convicted abuser, it was felt it would not be appropriate for them to take me on. I was further directed to contact another charity who specialised in working with, and providing funded therapy for, those with psychosexual problems, either who were having unsettling and uncomfortable thoughts, were actively viewing CSAM, those who had been convicted of either possessing or watching CSAM, and those convicted of contact offences. Following this, the charity (StopSO) funded 12 sessions, where I continued the work started in prison. The counsellor is a clinical specialist in neurodivergency and psychosexual therapy

The support and help, the clarity and understanding were way beyond anything I had ever experienced. The counsellor supported my diagnosis and helped me investigate and understand the other issues I experience that can be attributed to AuDhd. A great weight was lifted. I realised it was not my fault. I am not wrong. I just needed understanding, help and support.

On reflection

I understand (now, in hindsight), how my offence relates directly to my experiences and trauma as an individual with undiagnosed high functioning AuDhd. The serious mental health issues experienced by those individuals with AuDhd can't be supported unless the individual is aware that they are neurodivergent.

I think I was a ticking time bomb. Perhaps an earlier diagnosis might have stopped the sad spiral of self-loathing. Instead I might have come to understand and accept why I felt so different, why I didn't fit in with the standard expectations of behaviours, norms, conventions. I might have had support and help.

In regards to my offence, I carry deep regret and remorse. So many people were hurt as a consequence. Collateral damage to my victim's family, my family, people who cared for me. I *did not* commit my offence *because* I am AuDhd, but because I was undiagnosed throughout my life and didn't know how to ask for help or even describe my experiences and symptoms. I still made the choices I made. I am fully responsible. I cannot blame society or anyone or anything. Ignorance, fear and misunderstanding played the main part in my story.

I am now on licence. Doing very well. I have good support. I have my diagnosis. I have self-understanding and live my life as best I can with the knowledge I have.

I have continued my therapy. It will be a lifetime journey.

Author Index

Subject Index

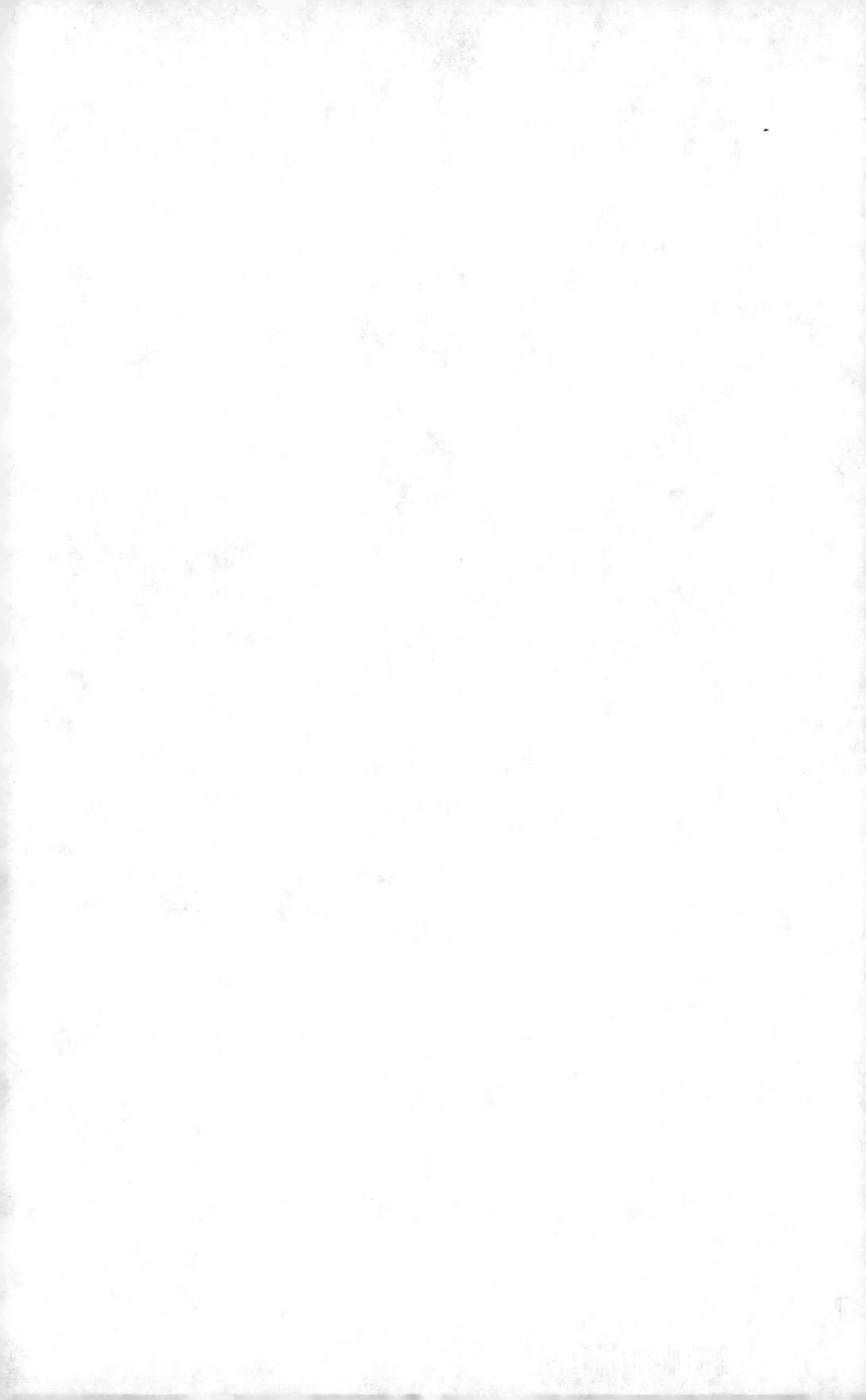

www.ingramcontent.com/pod-product-compliance
Lightning Source LLC
Chambersburg PA
CBHW050638280326
41932CB00015B/2702